THE AGELESS DIET

Your fountain of youth. The toolkit for optimal living.

TANIA VAN PELT

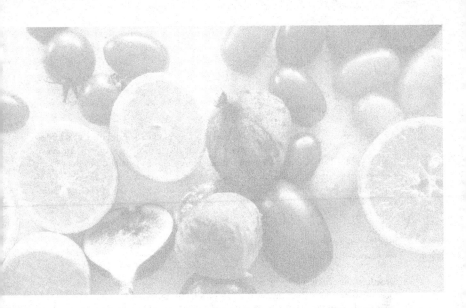

THE AGELESS DIET

Your fountain of youth. The toolkit for optimal living.

TANIA VAN PELT

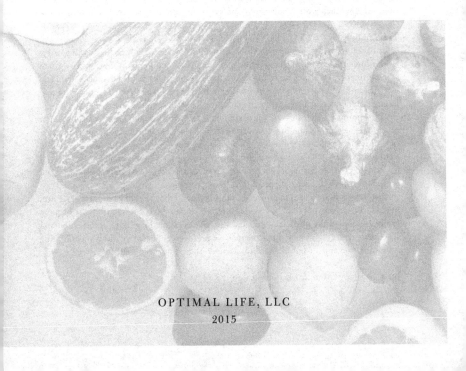

OPTIMAL LIFE, LLC
2015

Ordering Information:
Quantity sales. Special discounts are available on quantity purchases by corporations, associations, and others. For details, contact the publisher at the email address above.

Orders by U.S. trade bookstores and wholesalers. Please contact Optimal Life, LLC: Tel: (628) 400-3438 (DIET) or visit www.agelessdietlife.com.

Printed in the United States of America

Book design by Claudine Mansour Design

TABLE OF CONTENTS

THE AGELESS DIET

Your fountain of youth. The toolkit for optimal living.

TANIA VAN PELT

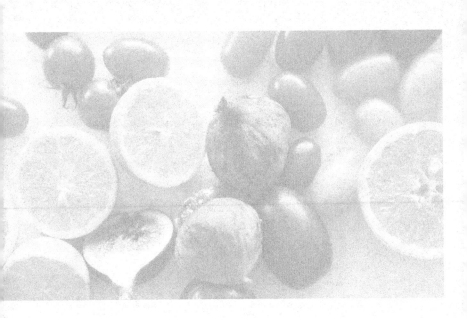

PART 1

The Basics

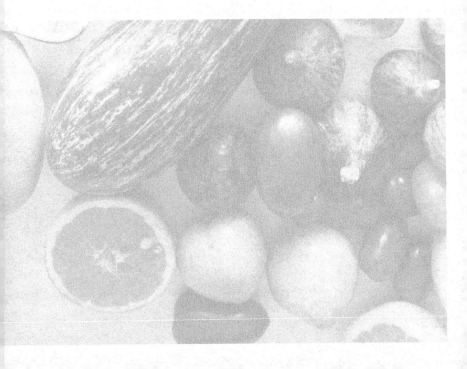

CHAPTER 1

WHAT'S IT ALL ABOUT?

*"As long as I am breathing,
in my eyes, I am just beginning."*
—CRISS JAMI

"It's the privilege of legends to be ageless."
—ANN WROE, author of *Orpheus: The Song of Life*

This book is your map to the fountain of youth. The toolkit for optimal living: 4 simple *Ageless Rules* to fix yourself on a cellular level for a younger and healthier you.

This lifestyle will cool down inflammation, help with weight loss, and stop premature aging. By making simple changes in the way you eat and live your life, you will rediscover the core YOU. It's also a more affordable way to live and eat, with a lower impact on our planet. Lose inflammation, stay healthy, feel great, save money, and help the planet by changing the way you eat? Yep. All of this is possible. (And, to make it even easier there's a support system available to you on AgelessDietLife.com with everything you'll need to become ageless.)

It's time we got back to basics—eating right, sleeping more, exercising daily, meditating, and having more fun. We are meant to feel good. And you will. All you need are the **4 Ageless Rules.**

Because of the cellular renewal I've experienced on the Ageless Diet, I think of aging as something different from getting older. I greet each birthday with gratitude. Growing older without the conventional aging makes each year a blessing.

I'm stronger, healthier, and more vital approaching my 40s than I ever was in my 20s. Thanks to my subpar lifestyle and diet my teens and 20s were far from the glory years. (I wish I could blame it all on being a late bloomer.) Poor diet and lifestyle choices meant that I frittered away years, and I wasted opportunities personally and professionally, because I lacked the energy and clarity of focus to grasp them. Let my decades of mistakes help you improve your life, starting today. You can begin by putting your health first. Don't punish yourself with a poor lifestyle. I've been there, done that, and it's definitely not the way to live life.

In high school in Virginia, I was just slightly above average. *And* I was no shining star in college. It's incredibly frustrating to look back and see those years squandered. College is usually such a ripe time for learning and experiencing, for freedom, and I didn't maximize this time. (You can bet I am now though.) No doubt this average life, wishing the days away, had something to do with my substandard lifestyle. In college my diet was beyond SAD (Standard American Diet, that is), and I barely exercised. (Did a walk to the car count as fitness?) I was desperately out of shape—I couldn't run around the block without getting winded—tired most of the time, and worried. Gone was the light, vibrant girl from childhood. Because my life was so solidly mediocre I looked forward to each birthday, nervously hoping that this year would be my year. The year luck would shine on me and I'd win an Oscar, become somebody. Never happened. Instead, some years were worse, some slightly better. It took me over a decade to realize that I wouldn't magically have a transformative year if I weren't willing to transform my lifestyle. I had no solid foundation from which to soar, to create, and to thrive.

My university diet was comprised of little dishes of sheet cake, soft-serve ice cream, some sort of dubious looking entrée, cereal with skim milk, and omelets at the dining hall, all-you-can-eat buffet at a fried chicken place, meal deal number three at my local fast food joint, vending machine candy and diet sodas, clove cigarettes, and six packs of cheap beer. That is, when I actually ate. The rest of the time I was too tired to put out the energy needed to forage for a meal. I had my version of the Standard American Diet, and the inevitable poor responses to the stressors in life. How could I manifest any sort greatness, how could I get even a little of what I wanted in my life, the love, success, and fun I craved, when what I was feeding myself created a sludgy brain and a doughy body? I was what I ate, and what I ate created what I thought, what I thought created my reality. And what I ate was crap. The worse I felt, the worse I treated myself. Rewarding myself with sleeping through classes, leading to loss of opportunities, eating shitty food, and choosing bad friends, who reinforced the feelings I had about myself. I suspect it was only thanks to the solid foundation of my childhood in South Carolina that I avoided eating disorders and bad boyfriends.

I had forgotten everything I learned from childhood: how to eat, move my body through space with exuberance, to play . . . how to live with joy.

Finally though, better late than never, I remembered what I had forgotten. I remembered how good I feel when I move my body and the clarity that comes from eating delicious wholesome food. And I remembered to set myself up for happiness with better food, good friends, and yoga. With each year since creating this ageless lifestyle, I am better. I am stronger emotionally, intellectually, and physically. I feel more alive and I look like the best version of me. I am happier, healthier, stronger and better looking now (I am better looking now) than I was on the cusp of 20. Those around me who have embraced the Ageless Diet are also more luminous, leaner, and live life with more energy. They feel reinvigorated even with the nonstop busyness of life—packed work schedules and on-going family responsibilities. It's a wonderful thing to be surrounded by positive, strong people. You can have this too. You attract what you are.

There is a natural fear of aging, of becoming obsolescent, ineffectual, and invisible. And, you're right, these things often happen, and they're awful. So, do we change our lifestyle? No, instead we worship youth, beauty, and the cult of thin. This is a sad irony because the majority of Americans are on the fast track to premature aging, inflammation-caused diseases, and obesity. Most of America has become what we fear. This is a boon for cosmetics, weight-loss, and pharmaceutical companies, and for manufacturers of highly processed low-fat, high-protein, gluten-free faddish foods. Shake lose the fear, skip the diet drugs and foods, the surgeries, and the fads, and take your life back by choosing the simpler, easier road. Transform how you feel about YOU by changing your habits. Become fearless at any age by taking action.

Growing old is nothing to fear. If we're lucky, it's inevitable. And you don't have to experience the deleterious effects of aging—cellular degeneration, weight gain, wrinkles, disease, weakening bones and muscles, loss of mental acuity and memory. When you feel good all the time, you can shift your focus to the benefits that come with age: greater wisdom, patience, acceptance, contentment, and compassion.

Yeah, yeah, yeah, you think, "But I still don't want to get old, and I really don't want to look old." Neither do I! As I approach middle age, I don't want to look middle-aged. I don't want to look like our grandparents' idea of 35, 40, 55, and beyond. I want the opposite: I want to be stronger, livelier, and more luminous with each year. I believe this is possible. This is not some crazy fairytale wish. With a great diet and a lifestyle that supports a naturally positive, gratitude-filled outlook on life, I believe agelessness until the day we die is attainable.

A diet is a map to the fountain of youth? Yes, and this book full of why it is and how to discover your own inner agelessness.

You might be thinking, "If diet is really the answer then why don't I feel great. I think I'm eating right, *everything in moderation,* and I still can't change my body. I can't lose the weight. I'm overstressed, tired all the time, and I can't sleep." Welcome to this American Life. That's almost everyone I know in New York. Even if you have a good diet and a relatively healthy lifestyle, they could be tweaked. Like me, in the beginning of this ageless quest, you're probably 80 percent there. It's the 20 percent sabotaging you.

Trillions are spent convincing us that real food comes in a package. Broccoli has no press agent. It's not our fault many of us have gotten fatter, sicker, and prematurely old. It's hard to combat conventional wisdom: everything in moderation. And ALL the money spent convincing us that what we really need to be healthy and thin is more of their processed products, more surgeries, more drugs. How can you get ahead if you've been conditioned to reward yourself with poison?

Two of our issues with aging are fear and blind acceptance. We fear the inevitable decline and miserably accept that getting older means losing. Losing our looks, our minds, our bodies, and our freedoms. And it means getting fatter in the butt and gut, sicker, sleeping less, forgetting our past, and having trouble navigating the future. Aging is all about loss. That's just the deal. It's how life is, after our 30s each year is worse, and each year we gain another 10 pounds. And, if you have diabetes, dementia, arthritis, high blood pressure, heart disease, and any of those other inflammatory diseases, you take your meds and deal with the side effects, right? That's just how it is. There is no cure for aging. We get old, we get sick, and then we die.

Yeah, I don't think so. Like the Standard American Diet, I'm not buying it. Not anymore. Those trillions of dollars are being wasted on me because I'm not buying the conventional wisdom, and the lies advertisers and big name companies are selling. I don't want to age predictably, the usual, accepted way; I don't want to be sicker and bigger each year. It shouldn't be a given that this is what happens to us. It doesn't have to be this way. We don't have to be a sick, aging, overweight population destroying our world. Aging and disease are almost always caused by inflammation, and this chronic inflammation is mostly caused by things we can control: our diet, our environment, our lifestyle, how we process stress, how much sleep we get, how often we exercise . . . ALL THINGS YOU CAN CONTROL!!!

I'm going to mention inflammation dozens of times in this book, and before we get down to it, to the nitty-gritty of living ageless, let's discuss **what exactly is inflammation**. The word is derived from the Latin "inflammo," which means "I set alight, I ignite." And it's the body's way of protecting itself, by removing damaged cells, irritants, pathogens, and thus beginning the healing process. It works this way: when something harmful or irritating affects part of the body, there is a fairly immediate response to remove this irritant. The signs of inflammation and the symptoms, especially acute inflammation, mean the body is trying to heal itself. The inflammation around the infection is the body's appropriate answer; it's part of the immune response. But, what if the cause of inflammation in the whole body comes from your lifestyle? Inflammation can beget more inflammation, becoming chronic and self-perpetuating. And often more inflammation is created in response to the existing inflammation. The body's just doing its job. This type of inflammation is usually caused by something environmental, especially including diet and lifestyle, and it's this inflammation, the chronic kind, that will kill you. Carrying around excess weight, experiencing anxiety, breathing polluted air on a regular basis, smoking, lack of sleep, a conventional diet, lack of movement . . . all of these lead to chronic inflammation. And this inflammation leads to many, many diseases. The body takes care of you as best it can, but in order for it to function properly you need to take care of your body. You can cool down chronic inflammation triggered by our modern lifestyle and diet. And the most exciting thing is that it's not hard.

When I developed the Ageless Diet, I knew, for sure, that I didn't want to be younger. Been there, done that. I wouldn't go back in time to a younger age. This lifestyle is not about rolling back the clock. Well, it is if you are aging prematurely—fine lines and wrinkles, bloated and overweight. And if you're suffering from modern day age-related diseases, most of which are due to diet, stress, and environmental toxins. Then you will be turning back the clock! But, for me, I'll be happy to look my best at any age for the rest of my life. Me at my current age, healthy, revitalized, and ageless, is much more interesting than chasing 25 or even 35 forever.

I admit it: I created the Ageless Diet partly out of vanity. I wanted to look good and lose inflammation-related weight. But the other motivator was a love of food and a voracious appetite. I'm what people call a good eater. I love to eat. I like to think about dinner while I'm preparing breakfast. I'm passionate about cooking and eating mouth-watering meals—addicted to food magazines, cookbooks, and I really enjoy grocery shopping. And most of all I love food. Insanely flavorful, bright, rich, nourishing, satisfying food. For me this diet means I can feel great and eat food that tastes fantastic.

I have seen my grandparents, aunts and uncles, cousins, older friends, and even my younger friends age faster and look older than seems possible. No one thinks it's weird that people get sicker and fatter as the bell tolls year after year. People may think it sucks that kids today are sick with asthma, diabetes, and autoimmune diseases, and dangerously overweight, but there's never any real change. Not yet. But there can be. You can feel better today; you can help the children in your life be healthier, stronger, and happier. This diet and lifestyle is for everyone, not only the almost 40-year-old woman who wants to lose inflammation, look good, and feel better. This is a viable, achievable lifestyle for the whole family.

It's time we fixed what's broken. The government isn't going to do it. Your boss isn't going to show you how to be ageless. The teachers at school aren't going to teach your kids how to live for optimal wellness. It's up to us. We need to make the changes necessary to get well, for ourselves and the generations to come, and we can do it. It's crazy to think we're all simply going to get sicker, heavier, and prematurely old and not address it, not try to fix it. There has to be an easier way to live.

I wanted to create some sort of real-life fountain of youth, using tools available to me today. This is not science fiction, and I'm not crazy. The damage done on young and old bodies by a conventional diet, junk foods, pharmaceuticals, too little exercise and sleep, and too much stress is there for all to see. I've felt the damage in my own body! And I've felt the magic of a clean diet, a good night's sleep, and daily exercise.

I believe we are what we eat, and I believe we are what we think. How we eat changes how we feel, how we feel affects how we view ourselves, the world, everything. I knew by focusing on what I COULD control, that by changing the way I ate and lived, I could change how I look, feel, and think about myself, and my world would improve. And, by losing inflammation, I'd probably slim down. I just didn't realize how much!

Plus, I was tired of eating junk foods. I know they're easy, fast, and cheap, and available everywhere, but this food is unsatisfying on all levels. I wanted better food. Real, flavorful, whole foods, fresh fruits and vegetables, healthy fats, lean protein, legumes, whole grains, fresh herbs and spices. I knew I could heal myself through good food, by creating simple recipes, making food that nurtures me on all levels. But, I never wanted to feel deprived. I wanted abundance.

The other reason I wrote this book was because of Mitzi. I didn't want to age the way my beloved grandmother Mitzi did. A brilliant, warm, charismatic woman with an unmatched zest for life, Mitzi was plumper each year and middle-aged in her late-30s. Then at 70, she was struck down with Alzheimer's, hospitalized in a nursing home by 73, shrunk to the size of small sparrow, and dead at 77. Knowing now what I've learned through years of research, I think this tragic end to a great lady's life could have played out differently. There has to be another way.

I am so tired of everyone accepting poor health as a baseline— my father with his debilitating arthritis and sugar addiction, my friends with their type 2 diabetes and gout, and other family member with chronic digestive issues and painful migraines, another friend with his ailing Parkinson's afflicted mother, my girlfriend with her out-of-whack thyroid and raging insomnia, and so many other dear friends and family with serious health issues that are clearly linked to lifestyle choices. Everyone blindly accepting that feeling bad is part of being human, that gaining weight is unavoidable, and that aging is inevitable. Can the Ageless Diet cure Parkinson's? Well, what I can say is that there is enough research showing a direct link between inflammatory diseases, including Parkinson's, arthritis, and diabetes, and a Standard American Lifestyle to get me to alter my diet and lifestyle. I don't want any of my friends, my family, my husband Scott, his family, or you to deal with this sort of loss and painful decline, because it can be avoided. Let's choose another path. Let's take action. Let's save ourselves, and by doing so save this beautiful world we live in.

We need to be fearless. Let's revolutionize the way we think about ourselves, about aging, about the food we eat, and the way we live. What we focus on expands. Today's thoughts are tomorrow's body. What you think affects how you feel and how you feel affects your body. Stop settling and start eating a diet and living a life that supports a beautiful, vibrant, AGELESS You.

Manifest the life you want with simple actions: eat great-tasting, life-supporting foods; exercise, sleep, and meditate daily. *This is the Ageless Diet.*

Who am I and why am I qualified to give you these tools for a better life? I'm not a doctor. I'm not a nutritionist. I'm a regular person. I've only felt healthy twice in my life, when I was a child and for the past five years. I love food. I love it enough to devote years of my life learning about nutrition. I've spent long hours over the last few years researching and testing. In the end, any diet program I create must to be supportive AND achievable over a lifetime, with food that tastes better than good. Because, I want to eat meals that make me feel happy to be alive, otherwise what's the point of living longer?

I've become an expert in food that tastes great and fuels a body right because I'm obsessed and because I've studied it and lived it. I've done the work and made the mistakes. I have lived both ways. I've eaten fast food every day for months at a time, partied hard, smoked, and exercised as little as humanly possible resulting in wasted days, feeling lonely and bored. And I've lived a life filled purpose, joy, and abundance. What kind of life do you want?

I've studied how diet and a few changes in lifestyle can transform the way a person looks and feels. I've condensed what I've learned into four easy-to-follow rules. I've created a program that supports you. So you can make the changes needed for optimum health a permanent part of your life. It is all in this book.

I was lucky enough to grow up feeling the power of delicious, healthy food. And, I've been blessed to be around people who intuitively knew a lot about health and wellness. I grew up with them. They're my parents. The hippies.

CHAPTER 2

THE EARLY YEARS

*"Parents aren't the people you come from.
They're the people you want to be, when you grow up."*
—JODIE PICOULT

My mother and father are still good cooks, but they were their best and most inspired, *their most dedicated to food and home cooking*, when I was young, growing up in a small beach house in Windy Hill, along the coast of South Carolina. They weren't obsessed with food, but they were engaged with the growing, cooking, and eating of it. We always had a garden. We ate real all-natural foods because they tasted good, and it was cheaper to eat this way than buy prepared foods, junk foods, or fast foods. I grew up eating all whole foods with very little added sugars. It was just the way we ate. I didn't give it a thought, and I never argued with my parents about food. There was no kid's meal; there was only breakfast, lunch, and dinner. I wasn't a picky eater. It just wasn't an option. You ate what was cooked. And the food was perfect; there was no need to fight over chicken fingers and frozen pizza. I never, ever craved packaged foods that were marketed to kids. Mostly because we didn't have a TV, but also I didn't want the airy, tasteless, spongy white bread my friends ate because my sandwiches were made with home-baked whole wheat bread. I can still taste the sweet nuttiness of this bread. This was staff-of-life bread. The craving for crap came later, when my parents divorced, TV became a babysitter, and they both stopped devoting time and energy to cooking.

The Ageless Diet is simple because it's based on living the life I knew in those early, tender, magical years. I wanted to feel as good as I felt as a child. And I do. Thanks to my mother and father, who while far from perfect parents, did me this great and singular service. They fed me the best food I've ever eaten, until these past 5 years, when I learned to make it myself. The thing I remember most isn't how healthy our diet was but how good everything tasted! We all felt great, basically all the time. My brother Rama and I were never sick, had zero health or behavioral issues, and pretty much always woke up happy and smiling. This was lucky because we had no regular healthcare. We were too poor to go to a doctor. What we did have, though, was a plant-based diet rich in flavor and diversity. My parents were young, sure, but they were glowing and radiant. And it wasn't the glow of youth—look at today's prematurely aging young—it was the halo of a healthy diet and lifestyle. I had boundless energy, so much fun, and a zest for learning, living, and exploring. I literally believed I could soar. Before you think I grew up in a Disney fantasy, you should know that my parents weren't happily married. We didn't necessarily have a stable home life in many, many ways, and we definitely didn't have a lot of resources. We were, in fact, food stamps poor. But what we lacked in income was more than made up for with great food and freedom to play. What we ate was a diet that today would be considered exemplary. Lots of superfoods, dark leafy vegetables, whole grains, anti-inflammatory spices, plenty of fruits, freshly baked whole wheat breads, lentil soups, black bean tacos, buckwheat pancakes, watermelon, raw honey on the comb, popcorn with kelp (trust me, it's worth trying), and so much more. It was all so delicious.

I had young parents; they didn't know they were supposed to be helicoptering around me. Plus they both worked, so Rama and I had freedom to run down to the beach and swim all day, to ride our bikes miles and miles, to explore the woods around the beaches and marshes. I'm not saying you need to live like a kid and play all day, but wouldn't life be better if you could? At the very least, you can add a little fun to your daily life. And the easiest way to have more fun is to feel good. If you're feeding yourself high-energy food and all systems are a go, even a long workday can be filled with opportunities for fun. Infuse your life with the vibe of a healthy, happy kid running wild. Our recipe for happiness was simple: we ate organic homegrown food morning, noon, and night, and ran around all day, and then at night slept really deeply. There were no TVs, no computers, and no smart phones, just books at night and the occasional movies at theaters. (I have all those gadgets now, but I still keep the bedroom technology-free. More on how to create a better sleeping environment in later chapters.) I was, despite our rocky home life, 100 percent happy and ageless.

Sure, you say, you were young. Of course you felt ageless you were a little kid. Not so. In fact, the opposite is true these days. Today's youth are aging faster than their biological years. Childhood obesity is an epidemic. Consumption of processed, highly addictive food is through the roof, and consequently most people, kids included, are sick and are rapidly prematurely aging. Many in the current crop of kids are overweight, and some are dealing with serious health issues related to inflammation. After a decade or two of eating a Standard American Diet, having schedules packed with meetings and events that require sitting in the car for long distances, these kids look far older than their biological years. It's distressing. And, it's happening in my family. Children today have type 2 diabetes and are suffering strokes; they're having cardiac bypass surgeries by the time they're 25, all caused by poor diet and environmental stresses. One in three children are overweight. And with that weight gain comes a whole host of diseases and premature aging. So no, being young doesn't guarantee agelessness.

But I was. Until I joined the ranks of avid processed food consumers and suddenly became a picky eater. What a surprise. Six months with regular access to television, junk foods, fast food restaurants, and school cafeteria meals, and I was hooked. Rather quickly I was picky to the point of impossibility. Only certain kinds of lunchmeat would do—a pale pink, slightly slimy, very thin slice of antiseptic ham—and only one kind of sliced cheese with soft, cottony white bread suited my new palate. No more whole grains! I wanted honeyed, crisped bunches of oats in big bowls of cold milk. Milk! Another new thing. We suddenly had dairy in our diets, and lots of it. Then the migraines started, along with regular bouts of strep throat and sinus infections. But let's rewind, before all this, because I want to share what I remember from age 7 (the year my parents divorced) and before. Magical years. Year 8 was another golden year, even with my parents living separately and having less time for us. We still ate good food, we still had freedom to roam, and we still had a big green garden out back that supplied most of our food. The rest came from the local co-op and health food store. There was not a lot of added sugar, no big hunks of meat at every meal, and no dairy. It was all just really simple, really good food. I went to school, did a little homework, and played outside until it was dark. Dinner was always, by default, a locavore's seasonal fantasy. Boy, was it good.

These were my golden years, and until my early 30s, the best years of my life. I felt free, happy, and magical. I know now that my very excellent diet gave me the foundation and energy I needed to soar and explore. And my distracted parents gave me the freedom to play, bike around town, swim every day in the ocean, read books, and create the world I wanted.

By the time I was 9, we were eating a totally SAD and conventional diet. My dad worked full-time, had custody, and took care of us. My mom also worked full-time and helped out with caring for us, but she needed time and space. I think both of them were broken-hearted and too tired to put any effort into meal planning, shopping, or cooking. So we started to go out a lot more. Popcorn shrimp (battered and fried) with hush puppies, and sweet, creamy coleslaw at our local seafood restaurant, Outrigger's. Bacon cheeseburgers and gooey, cheesy bean burritos at Rosa Linda's with a side of fried ice cream. Sweet and sour battered and fried chicken at the Chinese place up the road with deep fried egg rolls. Pig pickin' pork sandwiches on soft, mushy rolls with store bought pies in bright, lurid colors, and teeth-jarring sweet tea. Grits, with pools of fake yellow butter, and biscuits drenched in more of it, toast with grape jelly, scrambled eggs, and pancakes with syrup at my dad's buddy's beachfront diner. Make your own sundaes at Jeanette's piled high the whipped cream, acid-red maraschino cherries, candied walnuts, chocolate chips, and lava flows of fudge. I had McDonald's much more often, fish filet sandwiches, hot apple pies, and ice-cold Cokes. We ate frozen pizza on my dad's poker nights, Hardees' bacon, egg, and cheese biscuits, and Krispy Kreme doughnuts, hot-off-the-conveyor-belt, glazed, filled with icing, and every other kind you can think of. (They would later become a fixture during my late-night prowling for food when I first learned to drive. Krispy Kreme and Taco Bell.) And we became addicted to these foods. Suddenly buckwheat pancakes with raw honey didn't taste so great. I wanted that oily, salty, super sweet taste coating my tongue. Both my mom and dad gave in to our demands for more junk foods because we clamored, begged, and nagged for them. Plus, they were hooked too.

Did I mention we finally got a TV? My father's company was taking off, and we had more money. I had a $10 allowance (spent each week in its entirety on candy, cupcakes, and ice cream), we had a bigger house, bigger grocery bills—thanks to all those processed foods Dad was buying—and, yes, a television. I was addicted to this new food before I even tried it, because of the advertising. The ads were so colorful, filled with happy music and smiling families eating food that looked kind of gross, glistening, and inappropriate. I even remember how strange it tasted at first. I thought it tasted "off," and I distinctly recall the artificial flavoring. The frozen pizza was really disgusting, with its orange, too-sweet tomato sauce and flecks of something that was once distantly related to oregano, topped with shredded clumps of what smelled like plastic cheese, on a crust that was both crunchy and stale. But I ate it anyway. I wanted to try everything, and I didn't want to be left out. Every friend I made post-parents' divorce ate this way. The first time I tried those frozen TV dinners, take-out pizzas, or even fast food, I had to work to finish the meal. They gave me screaming headaches. I couldn't put it together, as a child, that what I ate was harming me. I soldiered on because everyone was eating it, and I wanted to be like everyone else. And after a few tries I started to adapt, and my palate evolved to accommodate the taste of processed food. After a while, I would literally salivate when we walked into the door of a fast food joint. The smells triggered my desire, and I was ready to devour whatever I could get my little hands on.

Dairy and sugar and meat became staples in our family diet. My craving for sweets was so powerful that if we were out of the stuff, I would eat a bowl of butter and granulated sugar. That first year eating the way most Americans did I suffered from crazy vomit-inducing migraines. They would last all day, into the next morning, and finally the doctor put me on drugs. No one thought that perhaps changing my diet back to the old way would make a difference. Even if our doctor had considered that diet was the issue I would have resisted. I wanted that food. It was worth a 24-hour pain fest to eat bacon, egg, and cheese biscuits and glazed doughnuts. My brother, Rama, and I both got so many cavities those first years on the new (standard American) diet, we came to know our dentist's staff well enough they sent us Christmas gifts! But I was still a skinny kid mostly thanks to genetics and probably because I rode my bike everywhere and swam every day.

When I was 9 I broke my arm. Badly. I was playing at a neighbor's house, and we went outside to jump on the trampoline. This was highly illicit behavior. My father hated trampolines and thought anyone who had one in the backyard was a reckless parent. This particular trampoline was right next to a sharp, jagged tree stump. Getting off the trampoline, my feet got stuck in the springs, I tumbled to the ground, right onto the tree stump, arm first. Immediately, shock set in, my arm was in a totally different, unnatural position. I calmly walked down the street to our house. My father's face telegraphed to me how badly broken my arm was, but I still felt no pain. I was still numb with shock. Fast forward to a year of operations, hospital visits, and courses of antibiotics. Because resetting the arm correctly became a months long ordeal, I never thought about all the antibiotics I had to take post surgery to prevent possible infections. I'm so lucky I had good doctors, and I'm grateful for modern medicine, including those antibiotics. But, looking back, I'm beginning to understand how those antibiotics affected the health of my gut. Suddenly it seemed, I had toenail fungus. And then I started getting tonsillitis and strep throat all the time. Coupled with my poor, sugar-saturated diet, was the weakened immune system. All the beneficial bacteria in my gut had been wiped out, and this was back in the day before they encouraged probiotics. My diet did the rest. All the junk food I was allowed because I was sick and injured, stuck inside nursing my arm while everyone else was at the beach, killed whatever good bacteria was left. The toenail fungus came from yeast overgrowth. This overgrowth can be triggered by a number of things, including a high-sugar, high-fat, low-fiber diet, impaired immunity, and use of drugs like antibiotics. The eradication of all the beneficial bacteria in my gut also severely weakened my immune system, hence the tonsillitis, ear infections, and strep throat. I wonder how long it took for my microbiome to be restored. But, you understand, we didn't know our new lifestyle was so damaging. We couldn't imagine that corporations would actively promote unhealthy habits, or that government agencies would tacitly support these unhealthy habits with things like bad school lunches, a wonky food pyramid, and dubious industrial farming practices. No parent could believe that milk doesn't do a body good—weren't there studies supporting this claim? Why would a busy working mom doubt that those enriched, packaged foods weren't full of vitamins her kids needed? Those enriched cereals, breads, and breakfast shakes were easier to pick up at the store than harvesting naturally nutrient-rich food from a garden that needed constant tending, right? Plus, those ads said they had all little Johnny needed to get up and go. Anyway, once I started feeling bad on a regular basis, it was almost impossible to pinpoint what was making me feel this way. Was it the junk food, dairy, wheat, sugar, the stress of the divorce, the gut imbalance? Or was it all of the above?

Things got worse when we moved to Virginia. I was sad to be far away from my mom and our life by the beach. It was a hard time for me. I comforted myself with sweets and fast food. I began to explore cooking. I really enjoyed being in the kitchen, but by this time, our cupboards were stocked with sugary cereals, pancake and cake mixes, bottled salad dressings, margarine, and all the other stuff that most people had in their pantry. I cooked with what I had and cooked food that tasted like what it was made up of—processed pieces and parts and some fresh vegetables and meat. In the summers I went back down to South Carolina to be with my mother, and I had a summer job working with her at Latif's, a popular French bistro and bakery. It was here I learned more about cooking, from professional cooks. I learned about vinaigrettes, frittatas, and constructing really flavorful salads. I spent most of my time with the pastry chef, my mom, assisting her in making custards, French buttercream frosting, whipped-cream-topped strawberry cream puffs, chocolate-mousse-filled cakes, drenched in a dark chocolate shell, big, chunky cookies, rocky road brownies, cheesecakes, éclairs, and so much more. I was in sugar heaven. And, ironically, I was probably eating better than I did during the school year, partly because everything we made was with real butter, real chocolate, real, fresh foods, and because after a while you can only eat so many slices of cheesecake and blocks of Belgian chocolate until you crave a salad or a sandwich (on a freshly baked croissant). But still, the diet was hardly ideal. And, it kept Mom and me hooked on dairy and sugar. On days off, we'd go to our favorite fried-food restaurants, eat mocha-chip ice cream after, and leftover pastries from work. Still, I was working a lot and having fun. Being 13 wasn't all bad news, and I was strong and mostly healthy because we danced around the kitchen at work, laughing till we cried. The moral of the story: eat real food, learn to cook, and dance more.

By the time I was 17, when I hit puberty, my poor diet (candy for lunch, mint chocolate chip ice cream for an afterschool, post-track practice snack, and a sensible-ish dinner) was beginning to take its toll. I would have a headache every day by late afternoon. Cue the Excedrin popping. By college, I ate erratically, mostly sweets, and smoked as often as I drank a Diet Coke—about every 3 hours. And I never, ever exercised. I was still quite thin, though I had a little potbelly that would stay with me until my 30s, probably because I consumed so few calories. I often missed the dining hall hours because I was absent-minded. And when I did, I ate like I was training for a food-gorging contest. Mostly, though, it was a diet rich in Diet Cokes and chocolate peanut butter cups. I would forget to eat, and when I remembered it would be fast food, either on campus (Pizza Hut or Taco Bell sanctioned college meal plan fare) or off, and, if it was a late night, vending machine stuff. I was busy or tired. Mostly tired. I didn't do that well academically in school. Average to slightly below average. Wonder if what I ate had anything to do with that? I did, however, find time to party. I discovered smoking, drinking, and dancing at nightclubs. I went out a couple of nights a week. Still, maybe because I was still a teenager, I was thin and pretty in a sullen Goth girl way, with dull skin and a lackluster attitude. I was a skinny fat girl, soft, without any muscle tone. Except for those dance sessions at the clubs there was zero physical exercise in my daily life. I would sink into these blue moods that lasted until they didn't. I was the type of person back then who stuff happened to; I wasn't the one who made things happen. It really wasn't until my 30s, when my diet got back on track that I got really, truly happy again. I forgot for years that I'm a naturally happy person.

I wish I knew then what I know now. I would've done so well in college if I had exercised a little every day. Exercise benefits the brain and the body. It's effectively like taking a hit of Prozac or Ritalin. It's essential, and one of the simplest, best things to ease depression. When I was a kid, if I said I was bored, my dad yelled at me, "Go outside, ride your bike to the beach, do something or I'll give you something to clean." And so, wanting to avoid that fate worse than death—chores—I ran outside, hopped on my bike, and forgot to be bored. So, why did I forget this essential cure-all for boredom and depression? In college, when I was bored I would mope around or take a nap. Now, if I'm feeling bummed out, bored or uninspired, I go for a walk, exercise, or take a yoga class, and I feel better within an hour. But back then, in my late teens, I didn't move my body unless absolutely necessary. Sure, I walked around campus to the occasional class, sulked around more like. Oh wait, one time I did go for a run, and I couldn't even make it a block. That was it for another 2 years, and it was a far cry from my previous fitness level of a 5:30 minute mile in high school.

After college, at around 20, I was in a serious slump. It was ennui at an epic level. What was I going do with my so-called life? I had no clue, no system of support, and I had no energy. This lasted for about 6 months. I slept through most of the day. I ate a lot of junk foods—a *lot of fast food.* I would eat at a fast food joint once and then go back every day for a week. I would crave it. After 2 days in a row eating this way, I was addicted. And I'd get distracted, itchy even, at around 4:00 p.m. when I usually got my fix, a.k.a. my combo meal. Lack of movement and a steady diet of fast food—I was the original *Super Size Me!*—caught up with me. I put on weight; I got chubby. And *that* made me more depressed. I would complain to my mother about how fat I was getting, as 20-year-old self-obsessed girls will, and she finally said, "Tania, this is boring to talk about. Why don't you just go for a walk? Do something." After a few months of complaining *to myself about myself*, I finally did. I got angry enough to do something else, and this triggered forward movement. I started walking a mile on the beach. Every day. And, a few months later, even though I was still smoking, I started running again. By 22 it became easier to run than to stop running, and I gave up cigarettes. But we're looking at another long decade before I changed my troubled ways. Before I started eating better food.

Even though I intuitively knew how to eat right for health and happiness—we all do—I didn't know the why and the what. I forgot how much I remembered from those early years. I came to believe that non-fat yogurts, low-fat snack food, and fat-free fig bars would keep me as lean as the commercials promised. I certainly didn't know, beyond realizing that what I ate affected my weight, how important diet was to happiness.

I moved to Seattle to study acting and became a vegetarian. We were mostly vegetarians when I was a kid and I decided to go back to eating that way, but didn't care to remember how to be a savvy vegetarian. All those years eating conventional dairy, processed foods, and low-fat products, buying into what the marketers and advertisers were selling, made me stupid. And, of course, I still ate a lot of sugar. I worked in a dessert shop baking cookies and brownies, so that was a mainstay of my diet. I ate like most vegetarians in this country, boxed cereals, fruits, pastas, dairy, and of course, almost anything and everything with added sugar. I once had such a craving for sugar-crusted raisin bran that I ate a whole box in one sitting, bowl after bowl with skim milk. It was here I learned an important lesson, after spending the whole 3 hours in rehearsal with a huge, distended belly: limit myself to three bowls of cereal. I exercised almost daily, and I was almost a normal weight, just slightly above average. I got a lot of colds. I suffered from serious issues with allergies and my sinuses. I know now these colds and sinus infections were triggered by diet and lifestyle. But I was in my early 20s, and didn't have a lot of interest or curiosity in health and wellness. I wanted a thin, toned body, but I didn't know how to get it. Everything health-related seemed like work. I certainly didn't associate what I ate and how well I slept with my overall physical and mental health. At least I was moving my body. I had my own form of meditation, long walks up and down the hills of Seattle. I was getting smarter, slowly but surely.

When I moved to Charleston, South Carolina, I got a little healthier. I stayed a vegetarian, and I decided to take it to the next level, diet-wise, and go totally fat free, especially fat-free dairy. Fat-free yogurt, fat-free cereal, and skim milk. Black beans and rice cooked with no fat, topped with fat-free sour cream. No more sugar-filled cola or diet soda, at least, but lots of baguettes—they're fat free—with pickles, also fat free! And low-fat ice cream and frozen yogurt. I kept up with the exercising, every day. And I slept well, but I was often low energy. I practiced yoga weekly, but I never cleared my mind or meditated. It never occurred to me. Meditation was something I had heard of but figured happened in a distant land long, long ago, or down the block in the oily smelling apartment of the Hungarian stew-making, incense-burning, mildew-collecting photographer with a thing for my mom. I probably couldn't have breathed my way through a meditation anyway, with sinuses clogged thanks to my hearty consumption of sugar, wheat, and dairy. And though thin, I had a soft belly and flabby arms. In fact, if I waved at you my triceps would have waved with me. I walked everywhere and ran a few miles most days so that probably kept my legs long and strong. I did 500 sit-ups and never toned the abs. I was often hungry because I was eating boxes of Kashi, a no fat puffed rice cereal, with raisins and skim milk for breakfast and lunch. I ate a lot of food. The sheer volume was kind of overwhelming. As my mom said, feeding me was like raising a chicken. The boxes of Kashi were my chicken feed. The chicken and I were essentially eating the same cereal. I needed to eat; I was hungry. It's probably why I went wild at night and ate a lot of low-fat cherry chocolate chip frozen yogurt, adding more chocolate chips from a bag as I spooned each bite into my greedy mouth. I was living proof that you can successfully eat an almost fat-free diet and still carry around extra weight. Life wasn't much fun those days. I felt bored and uninspired. I'd start one screenplay only to leave it unfinished and begin another.

At 26, I went to acting school in New York. While there I decided to commit fully to the fat-free diet, especially since I wouldn't be cooking anymore. At least in Charleston, I cooked black beans with mustard greens, jalapeño peppers, garlic and onions, every night. I'm in New York, why cook?

Why I, the skeptic, believed the conventional wisdom that a low-fat diet, that usually goes hand-in-hand with a highly processed diet, was the best way to get thin is beyond me. The anecdotal evidence clearly didn't support the claims the ads made. It's one of the stupidest things I've ever believed. And, I've been the poster child for bone-headed teens and 20-somethings. My breakfast was a fat-free cranberry muffin from the bakery on Lexington Avenue and 88th Street. What fat free means is full o'sugar! Lunch break from school was two bagels and a Coca-Cola at the Chelsea Market. More fat-free sugar! The other, more seasoned New York actors would eat their quinoa salads with a lean protein on top. What's quinoa, I thought? Then, who cares? That salad is full of fat. I'm sticking with my fat-free bagels and cola. No wonder I was also always exhausted by afternoon. I had no energy to power through the evening and all the rehearsals and studying we needed to do. Another opportunity stymied by a bad diet. Another expensive lesson (acting schools are not cheap): Fuel your body with the wrong kind of food and you will never have the energy to accomplish what you want.

After a few years in New York, and a long trip to India, followed by the worst jet lag ever. I actually ran into a wall I was so out of it and almost broke my nose. I decided to start eating meat, figuring I was anemic. My diet became more varied. New York is a fabulous food town, and I finally I wanted to sample some of what was offered up. But I still embraced the diet of mostly low- to no-fat foods. And, I was a size bigger. I went from size 28 jeans to size 29. (Now, I'm between a size 26 and 27.) My moods would fluctuate, like my sleep patterns. Some nights I would sleep, and others, not so much. It was in New York that I started doing yoga daily, and running four times a week. I felt decent, but never amazing, probably because I was still eating a huge amount of sugar. City Bakery's low-fat cinnamon muffins, Whole Foods' vegan cookies the size of my face . . . well, you get the idea.

In my early 30s I fell in love with the Coloradan who would eventually become my husband and moved west for half the year, dividing my time between New York and Colorado. It was in Colorado that I changed my workout routine. After years of doing yoga every day, I started working out with weights. Wow, what a difference adding weights to a workout makes! (If you've never worked out with weights, I highly recommend it. Start with 3-5 pound weights in a workout twice a week.) I got toned but I still didn't lose weight.

Then, in 2009, I met Sheila Heylin, who started *Happiness Series* with me, and she told me that if I wanted to drop weight—inflammation—I needed to drop sugar from my diet. And she was right, giving up sugar was the best thing I could do for myself. I told her, as you'll tell me, that I didn't eat that much sugar. She was kind enough not to laugh in my face. Give it up, she said, and you'll realize how much sugar you actually eat. And I did. Even though I consumed very little sugar compared to most people, I still ate something sweet every day. I had the perfect diet of moderation: a chronic inflammation diet. It was all things in moderation, including breads, cheeses, and sweets. What I realized after giving up sugar totally is that even a small amount of added sugar "inflames" me. I was working out daily, using free weights five times a week, but it wasn't until I dropped sugar from my diet that my body really changed. That's when I went from a size 28 jean to a size 27. It's true what they say, abs are made in the kitchen. You can't exercise your way out of a bad diet. Before, I was eating 80 percent healthy foods. But the remaining 20 percent (the sugar, bread, chips, and cheese) was torpedoing the benefits of the 80 percent.

With the creation of *Happiness Series,* a website about finding happiness in everyday life, I thought I'd finally discover happiness for myself. But, it proved elusive. Still, I learned a great deal about meditation, exercise, and how to live a life that supports a healthier mind from our featured guests, writers, and from years of research. And then the light bulb moment: I couldn't meditate my way to happiness without the right diet. I rediscovered the healthy, life-sustaining, crazy-with-flavor food I devoured as a kid. I decided to get back to cooking and eating food I loved. It was a treat for me to prepare this type of food for myself, and for Scott, our friends, and family.

Luckily, I had wonderful guides in diet and wellness, among them Sheila and her mentor, chiropractor Dr. Martha Linn. Sheila had done the work on how to live for a better now and a brighter future. She, among others, reminded me of what I forgotten—that by taking responsibility for my eating and tweaking my lifestyle and diet a little I could look and feel better. Sheila turned me on to meditation too. I discovered firsthand why a daily meditation practice makes an enormous difference in life. And working with excellent naturopathic doctors, including Dr. Carrie Louise Daenell and Dr. Paul Gannon, I learned all about vitamin and mineral supplements, how they can support a healthy diet, amplifying the positive. I learned from all these friends, experts, and guides, and I shared with them what I knew—how easy it is to cook healthy food that tastes great. This is one of those sadly well-kept secrets. Cooking is dead simple. And cooking good food is even easier. Start with the best, freshest ingredients available, prepare them simply, season with salt and pepper, maybe a little lemon juice, and enjoy.

I feel great now, but I spent years wondering what was wrong. Thanks to Sheila, Martha, yoga teachers, spiritual leaders, naturopathic doctors, integrative health experts, excellent home cooks, and all the talented chefs I've worked with through the years in the restaurant business, I was ready to create this Ageless Diet. I remembered what I'd forgotten. I went back to my childhood for the answers. I knew everything I needed to know about how to be ageless by the time I was 7. And, I'm only tapping into what we all know to be true on some basic, essential level. Eating well, eating healthfully, is part of our collective unconscious.

CHAPTER 3

WHY GO FULL AGELESS DIET?

Your body will be around a lot longer than an expensive handbag, invest in it.

"Let food be thy medicine and medicine be thy food."

—HIPPOCRATES

You can turn it all around, you can heal yourself, even if—especially if—you've lived a seriously inflammatory lifestyle. I've been there, and I've turned my life around. Helping you change your life is why I created the Ageless Diet.

Because I wanted to feel better than just ok, I wanted to feel great. And, I don't want to just get by; I want to succeed. I want to feel more alive, more vibrant for many decades to come. And, it's important to me that what I eat tastes really, really good on every level.

This is not a diet; it's a lifestyle. I wouldn't be able to stick to any diet that required me to actually *diet*. Because, as we all know, diets don't work. This is a diet in the old school sense of the word. It's how you live your life. This is not an exercise in deprivation, a no fat/no taste/no options diet; this is a framework for LIVING, for thriving. My goal is to give you the tools you need to create a lifestyle that works for you and with you, as it's worked for me and countless others so far.

I lived 80 percent healthy and felt way less than 100 percent, and I know when it comes to diet you need to go *all the way*, the full

100 percent, to really feel and look great. A diet of moderation will get you diabetes, fine lines, wrinkles, and the bonus gift of an extra few pounds added every year.

A few years ago people would often comment on how healthily I ate. And I did eat *mostly* healthy foods. But it was that 20 percent that kept me from looking great. With meditation, exercise, and a sugar-free diet, my moods were even, and I even stopped complaining. I found so much to be grateful for every day. My life hadn't shifted that dramatically, *my perspective had.*

Besides dropping sugar and finally losing inflammation, I started to meditate. *Finally*, I got it. Everything began to fall into place. 2009 was the beginning of my most fertile years, creatively, to date. Life is so much more fun when I feel good, exercise regularly, meditate daily, and eat clean.

It's easy to go the full go 100 percent because you'll be eating food that tastes so damn good. As one person put it, *"Ageless Diet has the yum factor."* Worried adding cooking, meditating, and exercising onto your already heavy plate of things to do will be the end of you? Don't be. The rewards you reap are exponential when you factor in the little bit of time spent cooking, meditating, exercising, sleeping well, etc. And, *this is your life*, what better thing to put positive energy and resources into than your health and wellbeing? You are worth it. What's the point of being alive if you can't do everything in your power—*just four simple things*—to feel great?

This book exists because I want to share with you what I've learned. And, I believe if we all feel better, we'll be kinder to ourselves and to the planet.

To feel great I dropped all sugar. I lost so much inflammation, I went down a full size, and my skin improved dramatically. I had more energy, more zest for life. My menstrual cycle was more regular, and my moods were better. I started to cook the food I ate when I was a kid. Scott and I felt like super heroes. We were at 90 percent. The missing piece was the lifestyle component.

See, I grew up with the ideal diet and lifestyle, and I've done everything wrong. I've had it both ways: I've felt great, and I've been sick and tired and depressed for decades. I knew the only way to feel and look my absolute best was to go back to those early days. With decades of cooking, learning and research I chose a single point of study. I attended integrative health conferences, read countless books and scientific studies, talked with doctors, naturopaths, nutritionists, fitness instructors and personal trainers, chefs, and great home cooks. And, I tested it. I started with the beta version on anyone willing to commit to the *6 Week Reset.*

I experimented on Scott and me first. He and I went full 100 percent Ageless Diet. Scott lost 42 pounds in 13 months; he was glowing from the inside out, instead of puffy and stressed. Like most of us in 2008 to 2012 he had very good reasons feel on edge and harassed. The financial and real estate markets had tanked, and he was scrambling to hold onto his company. But, he did the *6 Week Reset* and stuck with the lifestyle and he felt energized and looked the best he had since his mid-20s. Despite his imperiled work and diminishing bank account during those incredibly stressful 4 years of the Great Recession, he was doing all right.

I felt better too. Better than I had in a very long time. Consistently better, and not just that one good week out of the month, pre-pre-menstrual and post-menstrual I usually had. Because now I had the tools to feel good all the time, I had a support system that nourished me. The tools in my kit are the **4 Ageless Rules.** And as an added bonus, we stopped taking our daily meds, painkillers, decongestants, and antihistamines for aches, pains, and allergies. We didn't need those drugs to feel better because we lost the inflammation that led to the aches and pains.

Following these rules has enabled me to rely on myself, not outside forces, to feel better. My shift in perspective was all diet/lifestyle related. It was easier to shift my perspective about life when I took action, through eating right, exercising regularly, sleeping more, and meditating daily.

Choose your own health and happiness over financially supporting a well-funded, profit-driven industrial food and pharmaceutical drug complex designed to keep you hungry and sick.

What do I need to feel good? Kale smoothies. No joke. Meditation. Daily. Eight or more hours of sleep a night. Physical exercise. Targeted vitamin and mineral supplements to augment my diet. These simple things keep me strong, healthy, and happy. I had plenty of stresses in my life when I was young—parents divorcing, moving, few financial resources, separation from my mom—but none of them impacted my health and happiness significantly while my diet and lifestyle were right. I believe a large part of handling stress successfully is the way we live our daily lives. I ate the right foods; I had plenty of time to exercise and sleep. And that's what I'm doing now. I'm taking care of me, getting closer to ageless. If I feel ageless, I look ageless. And when I take care of me, I take care of others. The more I receive, the more I give. What I eat, how I eat, what I do to nourish my body and mind, changes my life, shifts my outlook, and I'm a kinder, happier person. It's amazing that a few changes in our diet can transform our lives, for good and for bad. It's such a simple thing, like trusting a gut instinct, we get suspicious of it, and we turn to pharmaceuticals, surgeries, doctors, and quasi-lifestyle gurus. But all we really need are four basic things: good food, sleep, time to meditate and exercise.

Even better, it was easy to implement these changes. Both Scott and I felt great, ate lustily, slept well, and worked with energy. We wasted less time, and worked smart versus hard. We both lost weight and have kept it off since.

As Katrien DuPlessis, a personal trainer and mother in South Africa, put it: "I was 42 when I met Tania and discovered her Ageless Diet. I made the decision to cut sugar from my diet, and added foods I've never tried. The best results I have ever seen. But most importantly the EASIEST way to achieve my goals of feeling better, with no more energy dips in the middle of the day, looking younger and more toned! I never feel deprived, I never feel hungry, and I eat constantly. Fruits, nuts, trying all the Ageless Diet recipes. The food tastes amazing, abundant in flavor, and I constantly feel satisfied. I have energy, my training is going superb, I have lost an inch around my waste and weigh what I weighed 15 years ago—even with muscle weight."

This approach to diet and lifestyle can be easily incorporated into your life, and you can do it without wasting time or money.

I've made every mistake you can make when it comes to living life and eating right. And because I've made all the mistakes possible, I know, learning through experience, guided now by research, we're all designed for exuberant living.

We are built for happiness.

It's possible and easy to start living a life that feels good at any age. Follow the *4 Rules*, do the *Reset* for 6 weeks and say hello to yourself.

After reading this book, EVEN if you don't make these changes in your life, I promise you will be more aware of what you eat, how you live, and what you think. And awareness brings positive change. One day, you will wake up to your life. For those who say, *"I don't have the time in my busy life to make these changes. And I don't have the money to spend on it."* Well, it takes a lot more time to feel bad, and it costs more to buy prepared and processed foods than it to shop for and cook real food. A conventional lifestyle will make you sick. Being sick is expensive and it wastes more time than you can imagine. We spend billions a year in lost workdays because people feel sick, over-stressed, and exhausted. It's because people are *inflamed.*

I'm confident about everything in this book. It's all been developed and tested through real experience. Test it for yourself, because the real answers are found in the *Ageless Rules*. Following them will allow you to experience a greater, more powerful, and energized you. It will allow you to be more fully YOU. I'm serious about helping you change your life, and if you want to transform yourself and your life you'll need to overcome your resistance. Because this is where it really matters, and it's up to you; it's time to fight back, to do what's right, what's best for you. Here's where you can really change your world.

Do the *Ageless Diet* for the next 6 weeks and *reset your body*, because you are worth the effort.

CHAPTER 4

THIS IS YOUR LIFE, TAKE RESPONSIBILITY, AND MAKE THE RIGHT CHANGES

"The price of greatness is responsibility."
WINSTON S. CHURCHILL

This is your life. You are responsible for how you feel, but it's hard to know what to do to be healthy. There's enough misinformation out there about diet to fill a hundred libraries. My hope is that this book will help you take control of how you feel and how you look. Greatness means owning your life.

Committing to the *6 Week Reset* depends on you, because no one else is responsible for your body and your health. The buck stops with you. If you want your life to transform you will have to change the habits that don't support you. Make it fun! Cooking can be a wonderfully enriching experience, shopping for fresh food is a privilege, exercising is a mood booster, and sleeping well is a necessity that requires time and space created by you.

You can't delegate your body's health to anyone else. You are the only one who can change how you feel, how you look, and how you age.

Remember everyone has an agenda. Companies that make food want you to buy their products, diet companies want you to keep dieting forever, and pharmaceutical companies want you to ask your doctor about taking their drugs. These are profit driven companies who spend billions advertising their wares. Their sole goal is get you to buy what they're selling. That's their agenda. They don't care if you feel badly; they don't care if you get sick and prematurely old. They have but one agenda: to get your money. You need to have an agenda as well. Your agenda is to commit to improving and sustaining your overall health and wellness.

I can tell you what rules to follow; they are simple and there are only four. I can give you recipes for healthy food with the "yum factor." I can share workout videos and guided meditations to use. But I can't make you do any of it. I hope you will. I hope you want to put your health and that of your family's first. But it's up to you. How you feel is UP TO YOU. You are now both powerful and accountable going forward.

There are a few things to do today:

1. Think about what you put in your body. Care about what you eat.

If you want to heal your body, you need to care about what you eat. Plan ahead, think about what you'll be cooking and eating for the next few days. Yes, it's a little bit of work, and requires foresight, but it pays off on those busy days. Find recipes that are ageless-approved, for dishes you can comfortably prepare and eat regularly. Stick to a mostly plant-based diet. A diet with some whole grains and seeds, legumes, and lots of fresh vegetables and fruits. Eat sustainably, for you and the planet. Move away from deprivation dieting. We all love food. It's a deep pleasure in life to eat flavorful, nourishing food. Change your focus from the idea of elimination—no fat, no starches, and no carbohydrates—to something that is bigger and more exciting, a diet rich in flavor, nutrients, healthy fats, and fresh food. And cook. Start doing some simple food preparation and cooking.

2. Detox gently, drop the toxic food from your diet.

Skip the harsh cleansing fast and simply start with dropping all fake foods from your diet. These include processed and manufactured foods, fast foods, foods with artificial flavorings, colorings, preservatives, and additives, processed and refined white and whole-wheat flour, white sugar, high-fructose corn syrup (HFCS) or glucose-fructose syrup, and all trans fats. Shop smart and eat clean. No more prepared foods, no more processed foods, no more food and drinks with added sugar. Throw out or give away all junk foods, all processed, sugar-filled foods in your house. If it's not around, you won't eat it. But make sure to surround yourself with food you will enjoy, food that energizes. Take apples, oranges, and nuts with you so you won't make bad choices when desperate from hunger.

3. Eat food you love.
Make a list of all the fruits, vegetables, legumes, lean proteins, grains, and seeds you love and search out recipes (AgelessDietLife. com is a great source for this) with the foods you enjoy most.

4. Practice Food Accountability.
What does this mean? It means taking responsibility for your food choices. I promise you your body already holds you accountable for your choices. Personal accountability is about taking responsibility for your actions and choices in your environment. Rather than blaming outside sources, seek to understand your role in every situation. What dictates your choice to eat poorly? Why is eating poorly a "reward"? Why do you eat sugar? Are you craving it because you're hungry, bored, lonely, or sad? If it's any of these, address the why before you eat something or do something that causes you harm. Bottom line, if you care about how you feel and look, and how you age, then no excuses. Make the time to prepare and eat food that supports you. Build a life around what nourishes you: sleep, a clean diet, exercise, and meditation.

You're not alone, though. Yes, you are accountable for the food you eat and the way you feel, but I'm here to help you change your life and transform yourself into a healthy, vibrant, ageless person. In this book you have a toolkit to show you the way to eat and live for optimal wellness.

When it comes to accountability we also need to consider the impact our lifestyles have on the planet. This means eating more plants, less animals. Less protein, more healthy carbohydrates, and when you do eat animals—beef, lamb, chicken, pork, fish, and shrimp—source it wisely.

By taking responsibility for your health you decide what works for you. You discover the diet that makes you feel best. I hope it's also a diet that supports a healthy world and an ageless you. What you eat should taste good and it should definitely make you feel better. Always remember that when choosing how to live and what to eat.

And, make it easy on yourself: start the Ageless Diet right by getting rid of all junk food, sugar, dairy, and processed wheat in your kitchen, load up on fresh fruits and vegetables, lean, healthy proteins, whole grains, and good-for-you snacks. Have the right foods on hand so you can whip up quick and tasty meals in less than 15 minutes. If you don't have inflammatory foods, juices, sodas, and flavored drinks around, you won't eat or drink them.

CHAPTER 5

FEEL CHANGE FAST

"Your life does not get better by chance,
it gets better by change."
—Jim Rohn

Positive change happens fast. Make it happen for you, start with the *6 Week Reset*.

And, here's where things get really interesting: you can change how your genes express themselves. If you have a genetic predisposition to diabetes, asthma, obesity, heart disease, hypertension, dementia, obesity, cancer, you can control your expression of those genes by making four changes in your lifestyle. Start with diet. Genetic predisposition is less important than diet. There is an almost 95 percent chance that a good diet will reduce the genetic expression of a health problem.

Let's look at diabetes. A study in the 1980s by Dr. James Anderson at the University of Kentucky was done on diabetic patients using a low-fat, high-fiber, plant-based diet. He demonstrated that within three weeks type 1 diabetes participants could reduce insulin by 40 percent, and their cholesterol dropped by 30 percent. Type 2 diabetes is a lifestyle disease, often caused by high blood pressure, high cholesterol, and weight gain. It can be prevented.

This bit of the study is even more germane, given the current epidemic of type 2 diabetes and obesity in America. 24 out of 25 participants with type 2 diabetes were able to completely discontinue their insulin medication. That's huge. This is the magic diet can work. When it comes to change there can be resistance. It's natural. And this lifestyle I'm encouraging you to embrace may seem radical, but if you follow the 4 Rules within the first 3 weeks you will feel much better.

Let me tell you what happened to a few fellow Ageless Dieters and me. After the *Reset*, I got leaner but not significantly lighter. I think I only dropped about 4 pounds. I worked out regularly with free weights and added definition. And because muscles weigh more than fat, my weight loss wasn't as dramatic as my loss of inflammation and pant size. I was thin and flabby before the Ageless Diet, and after I was toned and lean. However, Scott, who at 6'4" weighed about 228 pounds, lost 42 pounds. Scott went from a size 36 in his jeans to a 33. He's naturally thin, but years of skipping meals and then gorging on inflammatory fast food and big dinners at steakhouses had given him a big belly. He was aging fast. He, like me, lost inflammation, so he looked leaner and felt energized, even before the bulk of the weight loss. By the end of the year, he was significantly lighter, and he looked younger. Both of us lost the lines on our face caused by inflammation, and our skin was brighter. My friend Blair lost about 23 pounds of extra weight, and he went down two full sizes. He looks great. Anna, a high flyer in the finance world of New York, dropped about 12 pounds and, like Blair, went down two dress sizes. A husband and wife filmmaking team, Chris and Lee-Ann, committed to the *6 Week Reset* last winter. Chris lost a significant amount of weight, about 30 pounds, and his eyesight improved dramatically.

From Chris: "Earlier this year I was introduced to a *Reset* diet by Tania Van Pelt. I liked the idea of a diet that was aimed at a healthier lifestyle and not at losing weight. The diet was supposed to be 6 weeks, but my wife Lee-Ann made me a deal, if I joined her on the diet for just the first 3 weeks, she would do all the food preparation. I was in, and now I am very glad I made that decision. After 3 weeks of no wheat, no sugar, no dairy, no preservatives, no hormones, no processed foods, I decided to continue and do all 6 weeks. That was almost 3 months ago, and now the diet has become a lifestyle. Why would I want to put any of that junk back into my body! Since starting the *Ageless Diet Reset* I feel more energetic and focused, and my ruddy and dry skin, especially on my face has improved. Instinctively, I know my body is in better shape for cutting out the above foods and additives. It was not as hard as I thought, partly because I didn't have to cut out everything I like, like most diets focused on weight loss. I still eat meat and chicken, but only grass-fed or free-range, and now that I am more involved in what I put in my body I have managed to find all kinds of goodies without all the additives and sugar. My newest discovery is raw pizza, as good as the pizza I ate pre-reset. After about 2 months on the Diet I noticed something unusual, I could read the ingredients on the backs of packages, and these are really small fonts. I wore reading glasses and could not do that for over 15 years, and suddenly my eyesight was improving. It's hard to say for sure which of the things I cut out of my diet helped my eyesight, but it's likely the sugar, or perhaps a combination of all of it. And finally, as a side bonus, I have so far lost 22 pounds without dieting—just eating better! Now that our film is done I'm looking forward to the rest of the Ageless Diet Lifestyle, and exercising and meditating."

Lee-Ann, like me, was more impressed with the loss of inflammation and her glowing skin than the weight loss. She dropped about 5 pounds off her already thin frame. For her, and for me, the best part was the feeling of lightness. Her colleagues on set kept asking if she had been to a spa. Chris and Lee-Ann started dropping weight and glowing from the inside out after the first 7 days on the *Cleanse/Reset*, which encouraged them to keep it up, even after the first 6 weeks.

As Lee-Ann says: "My husband and I started the Ageless Diet on the 12th of January. I started at 125 pounds, Chris started at 264 pounds. Chris has lost 30 pounds, effortlessly. Although, Tania and I try to get him to exercise, he has lost this weight just by the food he eats and doesn't eat anymore. I have lost only 5 pounds, but feel tighter and lighter and my stomach seems flatter, I think it was the wheat bloating me. My skin looks and feels great, softer and the pores seem smaller, I'm no longer using expensive serums. I sleep deeper and better. The most rapid results were seen and felt in the first 7 days as our bodies were getting rid of the sugar and preservatives we were unknowingly feeding it. Friends were saying I looked 'luminous, glowing, amazing.' Now, over 3 months later, learning what to stay away from and finding healthy substitutes, this has become a lifestyle, we no longer count the days that we're 'finished with the diet' so that we can eat cheesecake again, like with conventional diets. We're excited about discovering new products and new taste sensations. Chris used to drink 2 liters of full fat milk a day, a habit which would make me cringe, he was hooked on ready cooked grocery store chicken, corn chips and dips, now he drinks water and snacks on homemade popcorn. My eating habits were a little healthier, but I would never pass up the opportunity to have a croissant and cappuccino for breakfast and anything chocolate I was always game for. Now it's fruit for breakfast, or brown rice and soy milk, there are so many delicious recipes on Tania's website that I'm trying out and loving. The endless sugar-free, wheat-free, dairy-free desserts are what get me up in the morning, another day to try out another new recipe. This is the kick I needed to start new healthy habits, for life."

Recently, months after the *6 Week Reset* finished, Lee-Ann told me that they don't even think about it as a reset anymore. "It's just a way of life for us, and we're still going strong. We love the way we feel, and we like feeling more connected to the world through the food we eat. I've even taken up running. Something I haven't done in years!"

Transformation happens quickly. Eating ageless, you'll notice how much better you feel and look within a couple of weeks, maybe days. But, the other side of that coin means that when you eat conventionally you'll be shocked at how quickly it can all go downhill, and how badly you can feel from the wrong kinds of food. If I ate at my favorite fast food joint or visited one of those fabulous bakeries in New York, and ate a few cookies and cupcakes every day for the next week, the results would be apparent. I'd be bloated, inflamed, achy, tired, and my skin would be spotted with zits. Plus, I'd be hooked on the sugar, salt, fat, and preservatives.

When you eat inflammatory foods like sugar, conventional wheat, dairy, fast foods, processed and packaged foods, you're not only feeding your body poison, worse your brain is not getting the fuel it needs. This is the beginning of brain damage. When we eat right, we think more clearly. We make better decisions, and we're happier.

CHAPTER 6

EATING CLEAN SAVES YOU MONEY

*"To keep the body in good health is a duty, otherwise
we shall not be able to keep our mind strong and clear."*
—BUDDHA

There's a money myth out there about eating organic, healthy food. The myth is that it's expensive; organic food is for the rich. Real food is much more affordable, all day long, than processed food. Real food is not more expensive. In fact, it's much less expensive to eat a healthy dinner at home then go to a fast food chain and buy four meal deals. It's cheaper to buy fruits and vegetables than bags of chips, cookies, snacks, prepared meals, packaged foods, and frozen dinners. It's more affordable to eat a real lunch, cooked by you, than buy a food-like lunch in a cardboard box from the refrigerated section of your grocery store.

Fresh food, a clean diet, is not for the elite; it is for everyone. And the price of junk food is quite high when you factor in everything else. "The truth is that the 'value' and 'low prices' of cheap food that we see at the cash register, are not the whole story. We are paying today in our health and our taxes and our children will be paying tomorrow with a degraded environment, dirty water, decimated communities and jobs, and denigrated health," says Ellen Gustafson, co-founder of *Food Tank: The Food Think Tank.*

It's worth your best efforts to feed yourself and your family real, natural whole foods. The time has come to stop thinking of processed foods as the norm and to relearn how wonderful real food tastes. It's time to see food as an integral part of a meal and not as a single nutrient we have to consume. This is how these big producers of packaged and processed foods hook everyone, by convincing us we should consume a sugary yogurt because it's fortified with calcium, probiotics, and other vitamins. And they make it cheap. It's very seductive, this inexpensive food, fortified with so-called nutrients you urgently require. But, it's not fortified with anything you need, and it's not cheaper. Eat the rainbow of fruits and vegetables. Embrace a diet rich in whole grains, seeds, nuts, and legumes. Invest in an olive oil or coconut oil you like. And stay far away from those processed, packaged food products, even the ones in a health food store; they are designed to be addictive and insanely (chemically) flavorful. They're going to make you very fat and very sick. Once you're addicted to the ease of buying the pricier processed/prepared foods and drinks, and to the taste of this chemically enhanced junk, it's hard to stop. I've been there, and it took me years to get off the junk food teat. My advice: don't start, and if you have, quit. It's much easier to maintain good health and a healthy weight than to try and lose weight and get healthy in the first place.

I know it may seem hard to compete with those cheap value meals at fast food chains or the prepared foods at your local grocery store, but creating delicious, wholesome meals from real foods, mostly plants, is much more affordable and rewarding given the long-term health benefits. Americans spend over $147 billion per year to combat obesity-related and inflammatory-related illnesses—nearly 10 percent of our total healthcare spending.

"We are spending less than half as much of our incomes on food today than we did 40 years ago, but we spend three times as much on medical care," says family physician Joel Fuhrman, MD, author of the bestselling book *Eat to Live*. "Instead of buying good-quality, healthful food, we eat ourselves into chronic diseases that cost a fortune to control with drugs, and the drugs don't work very well and have side effects too." That makes the cheap value meal the most expensive meal you'll ever eat.

CHAPTER 7

EATING ORGANIC, COOKING OUR OWN FOOD

"Integrity food requires visceral participation from more people. A kitchen centric food culture—this is what we need to change our food culture. People need to learn to cook again. And celebrate seasonality—spiritually and emotionally it makes us realize that we are dependent on our nest. Enjoy the newness of things. Enjoy our dependency on the land. We can heal the planet one bite at a time."

—JOEL SALATIN, America's most famous farmer and author of *Folks, This Ain't Normal*; *You Can Farm*; and *Salad Bar Beef*.

Organic is a buzzy word right now. But, it's the label we're working with, and our choice is between organic and conventional. Certified organic is what I urge you to seek out. On all my recipes I recommend people buy and eat certified organic fruits, vegetables, legumes, and whole grains. It's important to me that I buy organic foods when available. The food often tastes better and has more nutrients. But if you are in a place where organic is not available, it's still better to eat fresh fruits and vegetables than not. Organic means free of pesticides and other toxins. And when you buy organic you support organic farming. A 2007 study out of Newcastle University in the United Kingdom proved that organic produce has more than 40 percent higher levels of some nutrients (including vitamin C, zinc, and iron) than conventionally grown produce. Another study in 2003 in the Journal of Agricultural and Food Chemistry showed that organically grown berries and corn contained 58 percent more polyphenols—those anti-inflammatory antioxidants that help prevent disease and keep you ageless—and up to 52 percent higher levels of vitamin C than conventionally grown corn and berries. One of the big reasons for higher nutrients in organically grown food is the soil. Alyson Mitchell, Ph.D., an associate professor of food science and technology at the University of California, Davis, and one of the study's lead authors says this about soil fertility: "With organic methods, the nitrogen present in composted soil is released slowly and therefore plants grow at a normal rate, with their nutrients in balance. Vegetables fertilized with conventional fertilizers grow very rapidly and allocate less energy to develop nutrients." If you can't always buy organic for pocketbook reasons or because it's not as available, go for local then. Supporting your local farmers by buying their produce means more nutrients. The less distance produce travels, the fresher it is, the more nutrient rich it will be.

Remember: You vote with your pocketbooks. You want more affordable, organic foods? Shop organic, and show the grocery stores there is a market for it. You want less pesticides and hormones and antibiotics in your food? Buy organic, grass-fed, pasture-raised, and let the food industries know what's important to you. It's one of the easiest ways we can change our food system for the better. The planet can't support the current system. We're killing ourselves, and the world we live in, with this current method of food production. It seems logical that poisons like pesticides, added hormones, and antibiotics, are inflammatory and bad for us. (When it comes to what to eat, choose real food; if it won't rot, it won't digest. And, you want food you can digest.)

What do pesticides do to us when we consume trace amounts of them in our food? Well, the research is not definitive but signs point to bad news for our health. Think about it, if the pesticides and insecticides used are effective, then it's probably not totally safe for human consumption. We're all living organisms, and what kills insects and pests will most likely affect us in a way that's not good for our health. Many chemicals used in pesticides affect the neurology of the insects and pests, inadvertently affecting the neurological function of children, too. A 2010 Harvard study showed that organophosphate pesticides—found in children's urine—may lead to ADHD. And worse, researchers from USC found that "those who lived within 500 meters of places where methyl bromide, captan and eight other organochlorine pesticides had been applied were more likely to have developed prostate cancer." Pesticides on food and in the environment are inflammatory, and inflammation leads to health issues like obesity and diabetes. There has been evidence from an important study pointing to a higher prevalence of obesity in the participants with high concentrations of a pesticide known as 2,5-dichlorophenol (2,5-DCP) in their urine. Scarily, 2,5-DCP is one of the most widely used pesticides on the globe. Robert Sargis, MD, PhD, shared his findings at the Endocrine Society's 94th Annual Meeting. He said that agricultural fungicide creates insulin resistance in fat cells. And, in 2011 the journal *Diabetes Care* published a piece stating that people with excess weight and high levels of organochlorine pesticides in their bodies had greater risk of becoming diabetic.

But it's not all bad news: there was another 2003 study in the Environmental Health Perspectives showing that all these dangerous side effects from pesticides can be reversed. The body is resilient. In this study, one group of kids was fed a diet that was 75 percent organic and another was fed one that was 75 percent conventional. The children's urine was measured for pesticides. The ones eating a conventional foods diet measured four times higher than the official safety limit. But after only a few days of being on a mostly organic diet, the group eating organic measured one sixth as many pesticides in the urine as before, and well within the safety limit. Changes in diet can be seen and felt quickly. Bottom line: we don't need anything added to our food, not pesticides, antibiotics, hormones, sugar, or processed fats. Assume anything added is a toxin, and stick to clean, unadulterated whole foods.

One of the easiest ways to ensure you're eating for optimal wellness is to cook your own food. And, it's been shown that people who cook for themselves are often healthier. It's time to discover how satisfying cooking can be. I know cooking may be daunting, but it can be a deep pleasure. Cooking is simply a series of steps, none of which are that difficult. It also connects you to your world in a way that is simple yet profound.

Fresh food and a clean diet are especially important for the kids in our lives. If we want to change the food culture, make it so the big corporations aren't dictating what our children eat, then the time has come to change the way we eat and cook. Let's step away from this idea of special food for children, the kid's menu, and go back to the way it was before the industrial food complex took hold of our diets. Go back to the time when kids ate what the adults were eating, absorbing the local, naturally healthy food culture of their community. Let's feed kids the food we want them to eat, not the food advertisers tell them they want to eat. The best way to shift the conversation from what kind of Happy Meal to get is to include children in the cooking process. Teach them to love the nourishing meals you enjoy by giving them the same good food you eat. If you're the parent or caregiver, remember, you are in charge of what they eat and their food education.

YOU'RE IN CHARGE OF YOUR HEALTH— THE RIGHT DIET HEALS

"Health is a state of complete harmony of the body, mind and spirit. When one is free from physical disabilities and mental distractions, the gates of the soul open."

—B.K.S. IYENGAR

YOU determine your own health. The big lie we all like to believe, because it lets us off the hook, is genetics determine health. While genetic predisposition accounts for a lot of how you are created, the triggers for disease activation can be influenced (turned off and on) by what you consume and how you process stress. You can eat (meditate, sleep, and exercise) your way out of most diseases. There is an almost 100 percent chance good diet and balanced lifestyle will heal almost all health problems. You can affect how your genes express themselves. Most of our chronic diseases, the ones we most associate with aging (Alzheimer's, cancer, arthritis, dementia, diabetes, and heart disease) are considered inevitable. They aren't. We can change the way we age. In fact, the single most important thing you can do to improve your health, and to stop premature aging, is change your diet. Making good choices in diet and lifestyle, especially eating well, meditating, exercising, sleeping enough, affects our ability to create the energy we need to be healthy. And the more energy we create, the healthier we are.

Almost everyone you know is aging prematurely. And it's accepted as business as usual. I should know, I was the queen of premature aging with my protein bars, sugary non-fat yogurt, jumbo muffins, vegan cookies, my late nights, and zero time for reflection. Looking back at my creative output, no wonder I was in a dead zone! I just assumed that's how I was supposed to feel. Pop a pill and hope the headache goes away, drink a few cups of coffee and pray to feel more awake, alive. I spent most days wishing them away, waiting for a better, bigger tomorrow. But it's a mistake to simply accept feeling tired, run-down, overweight, and depressed at 25 or 35 or any of the decades following. Premature aging should never be a given. In fact, the *only* thing we have to do to prevent this is protect our DNA from damage. And if damage does occur, repair it immediately.

How do we do this? Keep our telomeres long and happy.

What are Telomeres? Telomeres are tiny units of DNA at the end of each chromosome that can shorten each time every cell divides. We want long telomeres for an ageless look and feel. Their length is considered a marker of biological age and health. As you get older, they get shorter and shorter. From the University of Utah Health Sciences: "Telomeres have been compared with the plastic tips on shoelaces, because they keep chromosome ends from fraying and sticking to each other, which would destroy or scramble an organism's genetic information. Yet, each time a cell divides, the telomeres get shorter. When they get too short, the cell can no longer divide; it becomes inactive or 'senescent,' or it dies. This shortening process is associated with aging, cancer, and a higher risk of death. So telomeres also have been compared with a bomb fuse."

It's incredibly important to protect our DNA because accumulated DNA damage ages us. This is the primary goal of this Ageless Diet. And it's the underlying cause of most conditions that kill us, inflammatory diseases like cancer, Alzheimer's, arthritis, diabetes, dementia, and heart disease. From the University of California, Berkeley: "Telomeres allow cells to distinguish chromosome ends from broken DNA. If DNA is broken there are two options after the cell cycle is stopped: Repair or Death."

CHAPTER 9

THE BASICS

"If we are creating ourselves all the time, then it is never too late to begin creating the bodies we want instead of the ones we mistakenly assume we are stuck with."
—DEEPAK CHOPRA

The framework of the Ageless Diet is a *6 Week Reset* starting with *7-Day Cleanse*. We're going to give your immune system a super boost, give you greater focus and clarity in your life, while showing you how your body is interacting with the world around (and inside) it. Your skin will glow, and you'll learn how to THRIVE. While most Ageless Dieters have a noticeable energy surge within the first few days, after 7 days you'll feel the difference. Even better you'll feel empowered, balanced, and alive. Feeding yourself food that keeps you healthy and happy is easy if you plan ahead and the food tastes good. I have provided all of the tools to keep you inspired, including new recipes, targeted supplement support, workouts, and guided meditations, all available on AgelessDietLife.com.

The basics of the Ageless Diet:

• It's a lifestyle, not a diet. I'm giving you a toolkit to build the very best life you want and be the greatest person you can be.

• It is dead simple. **4 Ageless Rules**. Four integrative components that work together.

• It's an easy to stick with. You won't go hungry, you won't be exhausted, and you won't feel jittery or depressed. This *Reset* is not about deprivation or calorie counting.

You're going to eat with gusto. You'll feel good, about yourself and your life, and you'll have the tools to get what you want. If it works for someone like me, the skeptic, the one who's done everything wrong, I know it can work for you.

Here are the *Ageless Rules*:

1. Eat clean. *Start by dropping sugar, dairy, and wheat. Get rid of all processed foods in your diet today. Eat whole, organic, anti-inflammatory foods, and take supplements to support the diet.* The focus with Rule #1 is adding healthy nutrient dense foods into our diet while removing any inflammatory ones that age us, weigh us down, and keep us feeling stuck and tired. We're resetting our system so that we may fully understand what nourishes us.

2. Meditate. *12 minutes a day.* In our increasingly connected world it is more important than ever to take time away and reboot the brain daily. With guided meditations available on the site and easy how-to basics, meditation becomes something we can all do, easily, without wasting any money. Something that improves both our mental health and our problem solving abilities.

3. Exercise. *30 minutes a day, walk, run, dance, practice yoga, lift weights, bike, swim, move the body.* The focus with Rule #3 is to regain control over your body by resetting and transforming it through simple workouts you can do at home or at the gym. Regular exercise gives you the best antidepressant there is, along with reducing stress, oxygenating the blood and keeping the body limber.

4. Sleep. *Sleep 7–9 hours a night.* Sleep restores us to our best selves, keeping us strong and healthy. It's essential for an ageless body and mind. And with simple tips on how to get a good night's sleep it's easier than you think and more important than you may have been lead to believe.

Let these **4 Rules** help you transform your life. They will balance and harmonize your body, mind, and spirit. They will heal your body, ridding it of inflammation. And, when you take care of your body, you heal your brain.

An inflammatory diet (full of highly processed sugars, carbohydrates, and oils), lack of movement, and negative reactions to stress resulting in feelings of fear, anger and worry, all lead to constricted arteries and inflammation. And this inflammation is the cause of many of our modern diseases. Cancer, diabetes, heart disease, high blood pressure, Alzheimer's, even impotence and of course weight gain can all be linked to inflammation. Often the symptoms we feel—like depression, bloating, intestinal pain, migraines, dementia, and insomnia—are caused by something environmental. The exposome: where you live and work, how you live and work, and what you consume.

From the Centers for Disease Control and Prevention: The exposome is "the measure of all the exposures of an individual in a lifetime and how those exposures relate to health." This encompasses all the environmental exposures from conception onwards. The exposome affects our genetic expression and may be much more important in determining our health than our actual genome. Some scientists are even positing that 90 percent of our disease risks are due to differences in environment, *in the exposome*, than from our genes.

These days, in almost all cases, because of modern day diet and lifestyle, genetic predisposition to a disease means you will get it. But that doesn't have to be the case. You can change your genetic expression. This is kind of revolutionary. And, it means no more excuses. Fix what and the way you eat, and you feel dramatically better. Make a few small changes in the way you live your life, and the results are even more profound. A genetic predisposition to a disease is not a death sentence, rather it's a great excuse to clean up your life and start living for an *Ageless You*.

This book gives you the step-by-step tools to improve your life right now. How to eat right, which supplements to take and why they're important, why exercise matters, how to meditate, and tips on getting a full night's sleep.

What I hear most when people are confronted with a new diet plan, eating right as the doctor has ordered, or starting a fitness plan is: "Where do I start? HOW do I start?"

Here's how you start: *Commit to the Ageless Diet Reset/Cleanse for 6 weeks* and feel the difference in your life. My hope is you'll continue this program for the rest of your life. But, let's start with 6 weeks of eating clean, exercising, meditating, and sleeping at least 7 hours a night.

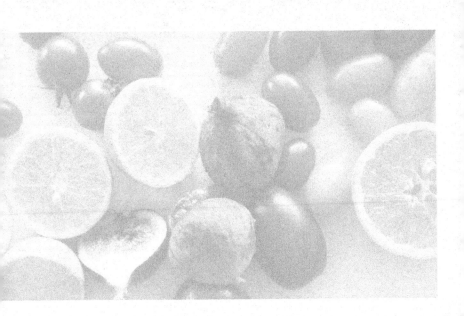

PART 2

Eat

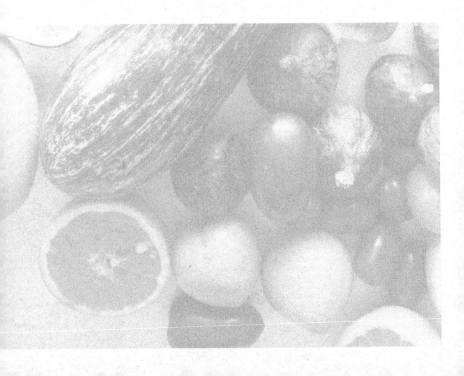

CHAPTER 10

WHY IS DIET THE FIRST AGELESS RULE?

"Health enters through the mouth."

—HUNZA PROVERB

This is the Ageless Diet, so let's start with the diet part of the equation: what and how to eat. The first Ageless Rule is pretty basic: Eat Clean Food. It's time to add healthy nutrient dense foods into our diet and drop the three big inflammatory foods that weigh us down, leave us sick, stuck, and tired. Real food heals as much as the wrong food harms.

So what do we eat? Plants! Dave Katz, M.D., from the Prevention Research Center at the Yale University School of Public Health, found that the healthiest diet is comprised of "preferentially minimally processed foods direct from nature and food made up of such ingredients, mostly plants, and in which animal foods are themselves the products, directly or ultimately, of pure plant foods." Basically, this means a mostly plant-based diet. I am for the 80/20 rule with my diet—80 percent plants, 20 percent pasture-raised or grass-fed animals.

Change your diet, and you can transform your life. Because what we eat affects every part of our lives.

With this in mind, I want to make it simple for you, and give you the information you need to eat right all the time.

CHAPTER 11

DROP THE 3 BIGGEST INFLAMMATORY FOODS

"Don't dig your grave with your own knife and fork."
—English Proverb

The Ageless Diet starts as a *6 Week Reset* because it takes that much time to create new habits and see and feel the positive effects from those new habits. For 6 weeks, you will be eating right, sleeping better, exercising, and meditating daily. After these first 6 weeks, you will have a clear sense of how this new lifestyle works for you, how the foods you are eating are really affecting you, and how you can incorporate it into your life with ease.

The first 7 days of the *6 Week Reset* is a *Cleanse.* Not a punishing cleanse of water and diuretics, but rather an easeful one that will actually clean you out and support your body's efforts to heal. You'll start your day with a power-packed smoothie, enjoy fortifying salads and lean proteins, complement your morning detox smoothie with an afternoon one, and savor a satisfying supper.

AND for the first 3 weeks, you're going to give up the three biggest inflammatory foods. *The top three foods that age you.* These foods are the biggest allergens for most people. After 21 days of eating a clean, anti-inflammatory diet, you'll be better able to notice which of these foods give you an actual allergic reaction and cause inflammation as you slowly, week by week reintroduce two of the three on the list back into your diet.

What are the top three inflammatory foods?

1. **Sugar.** Want to lose weight fast? Drop ALL added sugar from your diet today. No sugar for the full 6 weeks of the *Reset.* Zero!

2. **Dairy.** Give up all foods with dairy for the first 21 days. This includes cheese, milk, yogurt, kefir, cream, etc.

3. **Wheat.** Drop all foods with wheat for the first 28 days, including any and all foods containing gluten. However, you can enjoy gluten-free grains and seeds, including quinoa, amaranth, millet and buckwheat during these first 4 weeks.

Besides these three big guys, stop consuming *any and all processed foods.* This is huge. You must drop processed foods from your diet. They will kill you.

Dropping sugar means ALL SWEETNERS! Drop ALL added sugars, artificial sweeteners, and sugar substitutes for as long as you can. If you start this *Reset* by substituting one sweetener for another then there will be little change in your body, in your diet. Get the (sugar) monkey off your back! It is the single most inflammatory food for most people, and it leads to major health issues—in the brain and the body! In fact, just by dropping sugar from your diet you can lose serious weight and inflammation immediately, and see (and feel) real change within a few weeks.

After 21 days, you can add a little dairy back to your diet, but it's an inflammatory food for most so keep your consumption limited. Does dairy cause an allergic reaction in you? If so, drop it for good. I urge you to give up almost all dairy for longer than the initial 3 weeks. It's inflammatory in general, naturally high in estrogen, and very fattening (how do you think calves grow so quickly?). If you can't drop it entirely at least make sure the dairy you consume is 100 percent grass-fed and organic. Stick with grass-fed organic butter or ghee and, very occasionally organic cheeses, preferably goat milk cheese. Goat milk is easier for humans to digest. And bear in mind that most of the world—75 percent—has an allergy to dairy. Many, many more people are allergic to dairy than gluten! Do your best to avoid conventional dairy; it's poison, especially cow's milk. These cows are artificially impregnated for years at a time to keep them producing more and more milk; they only produce it when they have a calf to feed. They're also pumped full of hormones, antibiotics and other medications, which they pass on to you through their milk.

After 4 weeks, you can add back whole grains, provided gluten is not an allergen for you, this includes oats and sprouted breads. But continue to avoid all white breads and most conventional, commercial whole wheat breads with added sugars and preservatives.

Even after the *Cleanse,* for the full 6 weeks, drop any and all added sugars (not including naturally occurring sugars in fruits and vegetables). "Sugar is NOT just an empty calorie," says Nicolette Hahn Niman, author of *Righteous Porkchop.* It's toxic. This means empty calories are the least of our worries when it comes to sugar. Sugar causes serious inflammation, which leads to serious diseases and brain damage. It's so much easier to give it up altogether than to try to consume it in moderation. If I eat a little something sweet with added sugar, even in moderation, I'll want more later, and again more. And, I'm back on the sugar train. Consumption of moderate amounts of sugar regularly will prematurely age you. And if you don't care about this, what about this fact: sugar feeds cancer. Cut sugar out of your diet and you cut off an important food supply to the cancer cells in your body. In fact, dropping sugar is such a key part of the first Ageless Rule that the next two chapters are all about it.

CHAPTER 12

WHITE GOLD

"Sugar causes disease: unrelated to their calories
and unrelated to their attendant weight gain.
It's an independent primary risk factor."
—ROBERT LUSTIG, M.D.

The story of sugar ain't so sweet. But it is a compelling one. So interesting in fact books have been written about the sweet commodity, from how it Africanized the cane fields of the Caribbean via the slave trade to how it fueled the Industrial Revolution and turbo-charged the fast-food revolution. The history of sugar is full of tragedy, dread, and death, and that's before most of us got our sticky hands on it. Sugar was processed by prisoners of war, natives, and slaves at great cost to them, and then sold to the public, who greedily consumed it, making the demand greater and the public sicker. You could even argue the demand for sugar was the engine for the slave trade. "White Gold, as British colonists called it, brought millions of Africans to the Americas beginning in the early 16th-century. The history of every nation in the Caribbean, much of South America and parts of the Southern United States was forever shaped by sugar cane plantations started as cash crops by European superpowers. Profit from the sugar trade was so significant that it may have even helped America achieve independence from Great Britain," writes Heather Whipps in an article for *Live Science*.

It's a story of loss and more loss. We all lose with sugar. Sugar in all its deadly guises—the stuff that's in sodas, snacks from the vending machine, the packaged lunches from grocery stores, the school lunches, the deep fryer—is a leading cause of high rates of obesity, high blood pressure, diabetes, heart disease, depression, ADHD, and learning disabilities.

The history of sugar is a fascinating, dark tale. It was the Arabs who really finessed the process of refining sugar. "Wherever they went, the Arabs brought with them sugar, the product and the technology of its production," writes Sidney Mintz in *Sweetness and Power*. "Sugar, we are told, followed the Koran." Sugar is delicious and addictive, so where sugar went, consumption exploded. But sugar isn't easy to make. In fact it's brutal, awful work. I've heard from old Southerners when I was growing up in South Carolina that the hardest work they ever did was pick cotton and harvest sugar cane. The Arabs are the ones to really turn sugar refinement into an industry. From Rich Cohen's piece in *National Geographic*: "The heat of the fields, the flash of the scythes, the smoke of the boiling rooms, the crush of the mills. By 1500, with the demand for sugar surging, the work was considered suitable only for the lowest of laborers. Many of the field hands were prisoners of war, eastern Europeans captured when Muslim and Christian armies clashed. By the 18th century the marriage of sugar and slavery was complete. Every few years a new island—Puerto Rico, Trinidad— was colonized, cleared, and planted. When the natives died, the planters replaced them with African slaves. After the crop was harvested and milled, it was piled in the holds of ships and carried to London, Amsterdam, Paris, where it was traded for finished goods, which were brought to the west coast of Africa and traded for more slaves."

The more people tasted sugar, the more they wanted. The greater the demand for sugar, the greater the demand for cheap labor. "In 1700 the average Englishman consumed 4 pounds a year. In 1800 the common man ate 18 pounds of sugar. In 1870 that same sweet-toothed bloke was eating 47 pounds annually. Was he satisfied? Of course not! By 1900 he was up to 100 pounds a year. In that span of 30 years, world production of cane and beet sugar exploded from 2.8 million tons a year to 13 million plus. Today the average American consumes 77 pounds of added sugar annually, or more than 22 teaspoons of added sugar a day," writes Mr. Cohen. We're all addicted to sugar, but it seems especially tragic that the highest rates of obesity and inflammatory diseases impact the poorest of Americans, easy targets for the big companies to sell their cheap food to—food loaded with added sugar.

We weren't meant to eat sugar all the time, and yet it's in everything, and really hard to avoid. Sugar is designed to keep us hooked and make us fat. Sugar saves us in times of famine, but in regular, everyday life, it's killing us. The good news, once you drop it, most of the ill effects disappear. And once you stop eating the stuff regularly, after about 7 days, the cravings stop. This truth I can testify to. I've dropped sugar successfully and all longing for it disappeared.

If sugar is so bad for us why do we yearn for it? Well, because it can keep us alive. Sugar is a basic form of energy in food, and primates and then humans developed a sweet tooth to stave off starvation. Eating food high in fructose saved primates and humans when food was limited. But excessive sugar in the bloodstream is very bad news. Our bodies evolved to rapidly convert digested sugar in the bloodstream to fat. Our hunter-gatherer ancestors needed fat stored to be active during periods of food scarcity.

We have evolved to crave sugar, store it, and then use that stored fat when food is scarce. But sugar was rare, so we never needed to evolve to a world where every single product on the market had some sort of added sweetener in it.

And now it's everywhere, in everything, but we still have the same issue with sugar. We rapidly convert it to fat, and then we store that fat. Sugar used to be a rare and precious thing, good for saving us from a famine, but since it's cheap, readily available, and extremely addicting, our new issue is how to survive sugar. Our bodies were never equipped to handle heavy sugar consumption, it makes us very, very sick.

Added sugar includes cane and beet sugars, honey, maple syrup, coconut sugar, rice syrup, corn syrup, agave, stevia, xylitol, and all artificial sweeteners and sugar substitutes. All of these keep your body in a constant craving for more sugar and thus in an inflammatory state. Sugar used to be viewed as harmless empty calories, sans nutrients, but now we know it's so much worse than that. "The sugar is going to actually damage your body. It's not just that you're not going to get the nutrients," said Nicolette Hahn Niman, who learned this while researching her own book, *Righteous Porkchop*. At about the same time, the World Health Organization shared their study about the deleterious effects of sugar on the body and urged people to limit their intake of *added* sugars to five teaspoons a day (almost less sugar than in half a can of soda). But, given the addictiveness of sugar, five teaspoons of sugar is five too many.

Give up any and all added sugars in your diet, stop the inflammation and lose your addiction. Sugar inflames you and ages you. And the chronic inflammation that sugar causes leads to obesity, disease, and dementia.

As Lewis Cantley, director of the Cancer Center at Beth Israel Deaconess Medical Center at Harvard Medical School, said in *The New York Times* seminal article, *Is Sugar Toxic*, by Gary Taubes, "Sugar scares me." It scares me too. One sweet treat isn't worth the side effects.

Sugar makes you fat. Consuming added sugars, like sucrose and fructose, suppresses the hormone that tells your body you're full. "The title of a 2004 study says it all: 'Dietary fructose reduces circulating insulin and leptin, attenuates postprandial suppression of ghrelin, and increases triglycerides in women.' In other words, after you eat fructose, your body never gets the message, 'You've eaten enough, now stop.' As for those increased triglycerides, well . . . another word for triglyceride is 'fat,'" writes Jill Richardson, author of *Recipe for America: Why Our Food System is Broken and What We Can Do To Fix It.*

And what are fructose and sucrose? They are the carbohydrates that are commonly referred to as simple sugars. Easily digestible, fructose and sucrose can effortlessly enter your bloodstream and be quickly utilized for energy in your tissues. Both sucrose and fructose are very popular with the food industry and are quite often used as additives to sweeten food, enhance flavor, to make it so "you can't eat just one." But, as we know, excessive intake of sugar-sweetened foods, more than five teaspoons a day, can increase your blood tri-glyceride level, increase fat accumulation in your tissues, and raise your risk for developing type 2 diabetes. Sucrose, also called table sugar, beet sugar, or cane sugar, is the stuff used in baking cakes and cookies, and it's what people put in their coffee and tea. Sucrose is broken down into glucose plus fructose by an enzyme called su-crase, and those two sugars are absorbed into your bloodstream. Sucrose is half glucose and half fructose, and it is rapidly digested and converted into energy, and, of course, stored as fat for later use.

Just because added fructose in food is something to avoid doesn't mean you can't eat fruit, which has fructose. Fruit has fiber, and eating whole fruit is fine. It's the juice, without the fiber, that's full of sugar you digest quickly and store as fat. *The process of fructose absorption can be very rapid if the source of fructose is high-fructose corn syrup.* But, fructose absorption from fruits is less rapid because of the fiber and other phytonutrients in fruit. Fiber slows down the absorption of sugar, making a diet rich in fiber good for people with diabetes, and good for those of us wanting to be ageless. Eating fiber-rich fruit is fine on an Ageless Diet, especially low-glycemic fruits including berries, peaches, plums, nectarines, apricots, and oranges. Low-glycemic means these fruits cause only minor chang-es in your blood sugar levels. Yes to fruit, no to added sugar.

CHAPTER 13

DRUGS KILL?
SO DOES SUGAR.

"Sugar can cause premature aging."
—NANCY APPLETON, Ph.D and G.N. Jacobs,
author of *Suicide by Sugar*

You'll find after a week, you won't crave sugar, dairy, wheat, or processed foods. Your addictions will die. And you'll be feeling so good you won't want to go back to the old way of eating.
If I can do it, so can you.

I used to eat a ton of sugar. Probably, I have literally eaten over a ton of sugar. I was a cake and cookie whore. Pastries were my jam. But then so were candies, peanut butter cups, chocolates, caramels, sheet cakes from grocery stores, mint chocolate chip ice cream with extra chocolate chips added by me, and doughnuts, glazed, frosted, filled with custard, etc. So, I know how good sugar tastes, how addictive it is, and how it can stand in for the sweetness we feel we're missing in our lives. One overweight man at the gym, after complaining about not being able to lose weight and being told to drop sugar, said to me, "What's life worth if I can't eat sweets? I'll just do more cardio." There aren't enough cardio workouts he could do to stop the damage sugar does to his body, or the associated water weight it causes. My question is this: What's life worth if you keep eating sugar?

Back in the day, living in Seattle, I worked at a dessert shop, baking all day, popping chocolate chips in my mouth as I mixed the dough, skimming the tops of cakes for the frosting, eating cakes, cookies, bars, pies, ice cream, and ganaches. People used to say to me all the time, "Working here, you must get so tired of desserts." Were they crazy? There was never a day I didn't eat something with sugar. Never a time I didn't look forward to that first melt-in-my-mouth bite of velvety, buttery chocolate chip with a little dough clinging to it. Of course, I didn't quit. I ate sugar, butter, cream, flour, and chocolate every day I worked. And on my days off, I'd come and pick up the cakes and pastries that were a couple of days old and going to be tossed. *I never took a day off from sugar.* And for lunch, I'd walk across the street to the healthy, all-natural grocery store and buy a carrot, apple, ginger fruit juice and a peanut butter protein bar (basically a health-sanctioned candy bar). I can tell you I've never been asked out for dates more than when I worked at the bakery, even with a proper little potbelly. I swear it was the sugary aura surrounding me. These guys conflated the sugar they craved with the girl baking and selling it.

Drop sugar because it's highly addictive.

The thing about sugar is that the more you eat it, the more you *can eat.* Trust me, I know this firsthand. It's highly, highly addictive. Especially when combined with butterfat and white flour (a simple carbohydrate). It has been proven to be as insanely addictive as heroin or crack cocaine. This is not hyperbole. But unlike heroin it always gives you that sweet, first-time high every time. It ALWAYS tastes good.

I never maxed out. Sometimes, I'd intentionally eat to the point of nausea, just to make myself stop, but then when I was hungry again, a few hours later, I'd be back on that sugar train. And the rest of my diet included plenty of foods full of sugars, strawberry-vitamin C juice, those protein bars, pasta with a homemade tomato sauce, toast with sweetened, low-fat yogurt and apples, low-fat canned soup and a bagel with reduced fat cream cheese. I walked up and down a hill every day to get to work, and that probably saved me—the endless walks and my 22-year-old metabolism—from getting a lot bigger. But I couldn't, for the life of me, figure out how to get rid of my flabby tummy. Sit-ups never helped. Worse, I'd get these cysts. Even though I had naturally good skin, I'd occasionally have a really bad breakout on my face. They were caused by my sugary diet. I'm sharing my sugar-loving credentials with you because I want you to know that I KNOW how good sugar is. And I know how you can never get enough. But I also know how easy it is to kick the sugar habit.

The thing is, if you give it up 100 percent, you won't want it. As you may now believe given my past diet of sugar and more sugar, I have a bigger sweet tooth than anyone I've ever met, and now I no longer crave sugary sweets. Except if I haven't eaten all day, which is always a bad idea, because then I'll crave a big, fat piece of cake. But I don't. I drink a superfood smoothie instead. If you find yourself craving junk foods loaded with sugar, or are bored and wanting to eat something sweet to help pass the time, live by this rule when it comes to hunger: If you're not hungry enough to eat an apple, you're not really hungry.

Drop sugar because it's the worst thing you could eat.

Sugar is the single worst thing in a modern diet and processed junk foods come in a close second. Industrial farmed dairy is a very close third. The list of sweeteners to avoid includes agave, maple syrup, processed honey, brown sugar, corn syrup, high-fructose corn syrup, sorghum, molasses, cane sugar or syrup, beet sugar, brown rice syrup, xylitol, stevia, artificial sweeteners, sugar substitutes. And anything else you can think of that's sweet and added to food to make it sweeter.

Even those purported health drinks that everyone loves to spend money on, including kombucha and pressed fruit juices, they're not only high-priced, they're high in sugar. They taste good, because they're sweet, and we feel virtuous as we sip. But we're not that virtuous, are we? Juices, including pressed juices, are loaded with sugar. Sweet juices are basically just fructose, and have a similar effect on the body to soft drinks in terms of sugar.

Fruit juices and processed carbohydrates are typically high in sugar and enter the bloodstream quickly and raise triglycerides; this can increase your risk of heart attacks. Eating added sugars and processed foods subtract nutrients from the body and actually create nutritional deficiencies.

For those of you about to protest that you never, ever eat sweets, even if you're right, which I doubt, because we all eat way more sugary stuff than we think we do, you'll be surprised at how hard it is to find (packaged) foods that don't have added sugar. I'm not just talking about hyper-processed foods, check the labels on those little bags of crackers and savory treats at your local health food store. It may not be high-fructose corn syrup, but brown rice syrup counts. If you like dried cranberries, read the label on those: added sugar. Packaged Thai food, tomato sauces, ketchup, BBQ sauces, trail mixes, granola, cans of soup, pizza, hot dogs, frozen dinners, chips, biscuits, corn bread, bread in general, yogurt, cereals, most energy, protein, and food bars, certain brands of commercial mayonnaise, bottled salad dressings, and most "healthy" low-fat snacks all have added sugars.

Sugar is hidden in so many foods. Even in Japanese sushi rolls. Those caterpillar rolls everyone loves, because they're savory sweet, are loaded with added sugar. The eel in them is glazed in a sauce made of either corn syrup or simple syrup (sugar and water), with food coloring added. The sushi rice has sugar added to make it sticky. I know because I used to work in a Japanese restaurant and watched them make the rolls and the rice. And this was one of the better sushi restaurants in New York. Trust me, sugar is everywhere. I've seen sugar added to products that would never, ever need sugar in them: soy sauce, salsa, spice rubs, and cheese spreads. The point: sugar is in foods you would never expect it to be in. Most of us consider eating sushi a healthy alternative. It is, if you eat the way Japanese eat, less fish, more soy-based proteins, less sauces, more vegetables and fermented foods. When I worked at the dessert shop, the owner of the Thai place next door would sometimes come to borrow sugar. He brought a 10-quart container to borrow enough sugar to get them through the day. Americans, and now the rest of the world, prefer their food sweet too, even their savory food, so that's the palate he cooked for. I once had steamed kale at a resort in New Hampshire, and they added maple syrup. To make it taste better? I don't know why, it didn't, it was disgusting, but people ate mountains of it. We've been conditioned to expect our food to be sweet. Ask any European you know who has lived in America. They're always surprised at how sweet savory food is here, like those wheat crackers—sweeter than cookies some of them. And, tragically, we're exporting these tastes; people are getting sicker and fatter around the world. Their local food cultures that nourished them are dying, and they're poorer, fatter, and malnourished because of it.

Here's a short list, a general guide, on what to avoid:

- Soft drinks
- Fruit juices (apple juice has as much sugar as a candy bar)
- All processed foods
- Candies and sweets
- Baked goods
- Cereals
- Crackers and chips
- Corn products
- Fruits canned in syrup (eat only fresh or frozen organic fruits)
- Low-Fat or Diet Foods (to make this food palatable they often add a lot of sugar)
- Dried fruits (eat in moderation, and make sure they are unsweetened, stick with tart cherries if you want dried fruit, with no added sugars)
- Pasta sauces (most jarred and canned sauces have added sugar, make your own sauce, it's cheaper, almost as fast as opening a jar, and tastes 100 times better)
- Prepared and frozen meals (sweetener is most often added and they have other inflammatory additives and preservatives you would never want in your body)

- Sauces, in general (ketchups, salad dressings, BBQ sauces, teriyaki glazes, etc., etc.)

- Mayonnaise and Miracle Whip (check the ingredients on the jar)

- Peanut and other nut butters (corn syrup, honey, or sugar is often added)

- Jams, jellies, and other fruit spreads

And the list *does* goes on and on and on. Once you start reading all the labels you will be AMAZED at how many foods contain added sugar. We don't need the added sugar. It's inflammatory; it contains no nutrition.

It is also one of the most addictive things on the planet. Research shows that sugar can be as addictive as heroin or cocaine; this has been demonstrated by functional MRIs. In fact, a 2007 study, published in PLOS ONE, found that sugar gives your brain a reward greater than cocaine (title of study: *Intense Sweetness Surpasses Cocaine Reward*). Scary. And when you combine sugar with fat, as we often do in foods, you get something so highly addictive you'll keep eating it long after hunger abates. From the PLOS ONE study: "Overconsumption of sugar-dense foods or beverages is initially motivated by the pleasure of sweet taste and is often compared to drug addiction. . . . there are many biological commonalities between sweetened diets and drugs of abuse." What this means is that you will keep eating the same thing long after the initial craving goes away, because, as with heroin, the craving continues as long as it's fed. Stop eating sugar and you stop the cycle, not to mention the aging inflammation—*the inflammAGING.*

Added sugar in any form keeps you in an inflammatory state and wanting more, but sugar substitutes can be just as bad as the real thing. In fact, they can be worse because your brain doesn't get the signal it's had sugar, and the craving continues, stronger than if you had eaten real sugar. Sugar substitutes are also inflammatory, not to mention addictive. At least when you eat sugar you get a burst of energy, when you eat artificial or "natural" sweeteners (stevia, xylitol, etc.) there's no burst of energy. And you're left wanting. There's been nothing to deactivate that craving.

But what about stevia, the all-natural sugar substitute? "Stevia is 'sweet' on the palate, so the body assumes it's receiving sugar and primes itself to do so. Glucose is cleared from the bloodstream and blood sugars drop, but no *real* sugar/glucose is provided to the body to compensate [for the drop]. When this happens, adrenaline and cortisol surge to mobilize sugar from other sources (liver and muscle glycogen, or protein, or body tissue) to bring blood glucose back up," writes nutritionist Kate Skinner. It's this frequent release of the stress hormones, adrenaline and cortisol, in response to the (sugar or stevia-induced) hypoglycemia that damages the adrenal glands. These stress hormones are meant to be utilized in fight or flight situations, not from eating sugar, stevia or some other sweetener. Excess stress hormones mean a suppressed immune system, increased inflammation, and lower thyroid function. And bringing blood glucose up is an inflammatory response, causing, you guessed it, inflammation and premature aging. All this is at the expense of healthy skin, muscle mass, and immune function.

Drop sugar because it suppresses your immune system.

Sugar and sugar substitutes compromise immune function. They reduce the efficiency of white blood cells by 92 percent, and white blood cells are an integral part of your immune system. Each time you eat any kind of sugar it has the potential to reduce your body's defenses for 4 to 6 hours. Each time. Ever notice how you get sick after big holidays, after eating lots of sugary foods, too many inflammatory foods, and drinking too much booze, which turns to sugar in your body? The last time I was really sick—sick as a dog for weeks—was 3 years ago. Despite being sugar-free most of the year, I baked Christmas cookies every day for a week, and ate at least a half dozen every night. I got sick, sick, sick. It was awful. Now, when a flu comes my way, I stay even farther away from sugar (and orange juice!), I feel bad for half a day and then better by morning. Sugar weakens your immune system.

These sugar and sugar substitutes also overwork the pancreas and adrenal glands as they struggle to keep blood sugar levels in balance. When you eat something sweet it's absorbed into your bloodstream. This action puts your pancreas into overdrive, making insulin to normalize blood sugar levels. And it's this rapid release of insulin that causes a sudden drop in blood sugar. In reaction to all this, adrenal cortisol is stimulated to raise blood sugar back to normal. Keep eating sweet stuff, and it overworks and burns out normal pancreas and adrenal function, leading to early menopause, adult-onset diabetes, hypoglycemia, and chronic fatigue.

What about xylitol, the darling of health food store sugar substitutes? Surely, something from a birch tree can't be bad. Yes, xylitol can come from the xylan of birch trees, but manufactured xylitol most often comes from corn. It's much cheaper to make, and what do you think manufacturers look for when making xylitol? Cost cutting, that's what. The commercially available stuff is often produced by the industrialized process of sugar hydrogenation. This is from Sarah Pope, known online as the *Healthy Home Economist* and as the author of the book, *Get Your Fats Straight*: "In order to hydrogenate anything, a catalyst is needed, and in the case of xylitol, Raney nickel is used which is a powdered nickel-aluminum alloy. Can we say heavy metal residue? Most xylitol comes from GMO corn. Unless the label of a xylitol containing product specifically notes that it is from birch, beets or some other non-GMO source, run of the mill corn derived xylitol is very likely from genetically modified corn. This is the same problem as high-fructose corn syrup (HFCS) widely used in sodas and sports drinks. And it contributes to a gut imbalance."

A healthy gut is a healthy, happy you. Your gut is your second brain, which I discuss later, in Chapter 26. The microbiome each of us develops in our intestines—our gut—over the course of our lives is as much responsible for our personality and mental health as our brains are, not to mention our physical wellbeing. Some scientists want to classify the microbiome as an organ in and of itself because it has such a powerful effect on our overall health. And xylitol can mess with the beneficial microbes of the gut. The microbiome is now considered essential to good health, leading doctors and scientists to rethink the use of certain foods and substances that destroy the microbes. These include over prescribing antibiotics, consumption of processed foods, preservatives, additives, sugars, xylitol, and other sweeteners. Ms. Pope, from the same piece, continues, "Sugar alcohols like xylitol are not broken down in the stomach like other sweeteners. Rather, they arrive intact into the intestines. At that point, a process called 'passive diffusion' takes place whereby the xylitol draws water into the bowels. This results in only partial breakdown of the xylitol. The unmetabolized portion ferments; the perfect environment for undesirable bacteria to grow. This is exactly why consuming xylitol can make some folks so gassy and can even trigger cramping and diarrhea. Gut pathogens having a heyday in your intestines give off a lot of smelly toxins!"

Beneficial gut microbes help to control leakage through both the intestinal lining and the blood-brain barrier, which ordinarily protects the brain from potentially harmful agents. But feeding the gut foods that kill the beneficial microbes and foster the undesirable ones leads to all sorts of health issues.

The bottom line with sugar substitutes like xylitol and stevia is that at best they keep you craving sugar, at worst they disrupt your gut's delicate ecosystem, the microbiome. It's much easier to quit these sweeteners and other sugars than to consume a moderate amount here and there.

Avoid agave too. Agave has more fructose than high-fructose corn syrup.

Drop sugar because it leads to premature aging.

"We know that sweetness can increase the pleasure centers of the brain, the opioid centers," David Kessler, former FDA commissioner and author of *The End of Overeating: Taking Control of the Insatiable American Appetite* said. "We know it can serve as a mild pain relief. . . . I'm eating something that is sweet—it can change how I feel. So it's salient. It is powerful. It's directly hard-wired from our sensory receptors in our mouth to our brain. You don't even have to go through the bloodstream. It's a very powerful molecule because it's directly wired to our brain. And it can drive want. Add fat to that, it becomes more powerful. Add color, add texture, add temperature, add mouthfeel. Kids' candies are just very simple, but as you get older you want more levels of stimulation. But at the core of most foods that are hard to resist there is sweetness."

Why do you think they spend so much money developing these sugar-rich processed foods? Because the more you eat, the more money they make. Like the potato chip advertisement famously says, "You can't eat just one." Just like most of us probably couldn't do one line of cocaine. We would want more. Your brain builds up a tolerance to sugar, as it would with cigarettes, cocaine, and alcohol. The more you eat of sugar, the more you want, and the greater the chance of serious damage from chronic inflammation. Inflammation equals aging, dis-ease, bloating, weight gain, and so much more.

But never mind the addictiveness of sugar, consumption of natural and artificial sweeteners is aging. The reaction the body has to stevia, xylitol, high-fructose corn syrup, aspartame, beet sugar, cane syrup, agave, and their sugary colleagues is a stressful one. And that stress ages us.

Sugar is an anti-nutrient. What's an anti-nutrient? It takes nutrients from the body to process sugar; more nutrients are needed to fight the effects from sugar.

Sugar speeds up the aging process. Sugar overloads what's called the insulin pathway. And this overload affects your blood vessels and accelerates skin's aging process.

Give up the sweet stuff and you'll see a difference within one week. The change: clearer skin and more vibrant skin tone, less water weight, tighter body, and a more focused mind. Chris, the film producer, dropped sugar—and he loved it almost as much as he loved dairy —and his eyesight dramatically improved. His skin was smoother and less blotchy too. I lost 2 dress sizes, and my skin cleared up; I was glowing from the inside out.

Heart surgeon Dr. Dwight Lundell writes: "When we consume simple carbohydrates such as sugar, blood sugar rises rapidly. In response, the pancreas secretes insulin whose primary purpose is to drive sugar into each cell where it is stored for energy. If the cell is full and does not need glucose, it is rejected to avoid extra sugar gumming up the works. When the full cells reject the extra glucose, blood sugar rises producing more insulin and the glucose converts to stored fat. What does all this have to do with inflammation? Blood sugar is controlled in a very narrow range. Extra sugar molecules attach to a variety of proteins that in turn injure the blood vessel wall. This repeated injury to the blood vessel wall sets off inflammation. When you spike your blood sugar level several times a day, every day, it is exactly like taking sandpaper to the inside of your delicate blood vessels."

Drop sugar because it damages the brain.

A study published in *The New England Journal of Medicine* discovered that levels of blood sugar directly relate to risk for dementia. It found that even small elevations of blood sugar translated into a significant increased risk for dementia, even among people without diabetes.

Remember those overloaded insulin pathways? They negatively affect your blood vessels and accelerate the skin's aging process.

What about processed foods? Are they as poisonous as sugar? Hell, yes. For these next six weeks of the *Reset,* give up all processed foods. Foods rich in processed fats and sugars can supercharge the brain's reward system, which can overpower the brain's ability to tell an individual to stop eating.

Obese people aren't fat because they're lazy. They're overweight—*70 percent of America is fat*—in large part because the food sold is available in abundance, it's cheap, and engineered to be highly addictive, hyper inflammatory. Oh, and it causes brain damage.

Baked goods, chips, cookies, fast food, diet foods, junk foods, frozen dinners, boxed macaroni and cheese, sauces, dressings, condiments, pizzas, and almost all most packaged and prepared foods have added sweeteners, additives, artificial flavors, and chemicals to alter the food's textures. These are chemicals your body will never, ever need: factory-created fats, preservatives to give them long shelf lives, nitrates, hydrogenated oils, extra salt, pesticides, and additives that destroy all our good gut bacteria. And, in the process of manu-facturing these food-like substances all the nutrients stripped away. Antioxidants, soluble fiber, good, naturally occurring fats, they're all gone. Plus, they blow up our expectations for how food should taste. After a steady diet of frozen dinners, prepared foods from the grocery story, and pseudo-healthy treats, our palate dramatically changes. I know mine did. A fresh peach wasn't as good as peach flavored frozen yogurt. People become used to the taste of artificial strawberry flavoring, and it's sold at a fraction of the cost of an or-ganic strawberry, skewing expectations for what food should cost. We quit valuing real food. It becomes too expensive. These food-like meals and snacks change the way we view our world, and that has become incredibly destructive to our bodies and our planet.

Best things you can do to avoid added sugars and processed foods is cook, seek out lots of fresh produce, read labels, and retrain your palate to enjoy real, whole foods.

CHAPTER 14

DROP DAIRY

"Dairy is nature's perfect food—but only if you're a calf."
—Dr. Mark Hyman

Dairy is often promoted as a healthy way to eat more protein and an excellent way to get more calcium in your diet. It's also used as a flavoring agent in foods (processed and otherwise) and as a fat in cooking. The dairy industry in the United States is powerful, and they spend big bucks convincing us that milk does a body good because of the calcium and protein it provides. All this money spent on marketing can make the issue of whether dairy is healthy confusing. I want to keep things clear and simple for you, that means dispelling myths and confusion around food. Eating dairy is not the right way to get more protein and calcium in your diet.

Dairy has no fiber and no complex carbohydrates. It has less protein than most vegetables. It is saturated with fat and cholesterol (skim milk is not an answer, you're still consuming casein). Milk has no iron and blocks the absorption of iron from other sources. Dairy can result in insulin-dependent diabetes in the later years of life. And instead of preventing osteoporosis, dairy actually causes it. Chinese women who consume calcium from plant sources have lesser incidents of bone fractures in old age than their Western counterparts.

A study published in the *BMJ* (a weekly peer reviewed medical journal) suggests that high dairy intake doesn't protect against bone fracture and, worse, may in fact lead to increased mortality. Authors of the study showed that the high levels of the sugars lactose and galactose in milk may cause bones to undergo changes—like inflammation—that hastens aging and leads to fractures. Milk gives you brittle bones and brings on premature aging and increased likelihood of death. Studies done in animals, supplementing their diet with galactose (a sugar of the hexose class that is a constituent of lactose and many polysaccharides), increased aging processes caused chronic inflammation and oxidative stress, thereby rapidly accelerating the aging process.

Americans consume excessive amounts of dairy and animal protein. We are addicted. The savvy Dairy Industry has spent billions convincing us it is necessary for strong bones and a healthy body. If you think you need to eat and drink dairy for calcium, and because it's high in protein, think again. Animal proteins in meat and dairy metabolize to strong acids, unlike plant proteins. High acidity can lead to premature aging and disease. High acidity can make it hard to absorb the calcium and other nutrients you need. Plants, calorie-for-calorie, have more protein than beef. Dr. T. Colin Campbell of *The China Study* says milk proteins are the most powerful cancer drivers. And if something is cancer causing, you can bet it will age you.

If you're concerned about not getting enough calcium, because we do need calcium for a healthy body and good skin, don't worry. You'll get it from foods that are naturally high in calcium like fruits, vegetables, nuts, soybeans, oranges, celery, spinach, broccoli, kale, and almonds.

The most basic tenet of the first Ageless Rule is cleaning up our diet and subtracting foods that inflame and age us. Dairy is one of those foods for a great many people.

Eating ageless includes staying away from dairy for the first 3 weeks of the *Reset*. After the initial 21 days, you can test your body's allergic response to dairy by reintroducing a little. Be judicious, though, a little dairy goes a long way. And please stick with grass-fed, pasture-raised dairy. If you do have dairy, try goat milk, which is lower in lactose (milk sugars) and easier for humans to digest. Goat milk is closest in structure to human milk.

I found that after eating clean for the first 21 days, I was, *I am*, allergic to dairy. I can handle a little goat milk feta cheese here and there, but it's best for me if I limit my consumption of dairy. Before the *Reset*, I couldn't really figure out what I was actually allergic to because I was consuming so many different potential allergens; my body was in a constant state of inflammation. Was it the daily loaf of white bread? I don't know. Or the cookies and cakes I baked? Or what about the little bit of ice cream I ate every other day? Maybe it was the blocks of cheese, but I had no way of really knowing. This is why we eliminate all allergens in the beginning, especially for those first 7 days of *Cleanse* and *Reset*. For the rest of the 21 days, dairy is still off the menu. We're detoxing and resetting the body. This gives us a clean slate to discover what triggers inflammation in our bodies. I know, for sure, that sugar inflames us, as do processed foods. And, for many of us, so does dairy.

After my first 21 days on the *Reset*, I learned that dairy was congesting. Here's a tip: have a cold you can't shake, drop dairy, it's mucus producing. Dairy was also bad for my digestion. And, after giving it up for those first several weeks, I no longer craved it. I went from eating a huge hunk of cheese daily to substituting my dairy fix with hummus and other dips, and the urge to eat cheese disappeared. Since I reset my body and cleaned up my diet, I've learned I can handle a little dairy here and there, but my body is happier when I avoid the creamy, milky crack. The other issue for me is if I allow myself to have a chunk of cheddar while on vacation, it suddenly turns into a regular thing, and then after a few days I feel bad, congested, bloated, and heavy.

Quick sidebar about ghee, a cornerstone in the Indian and Ayurvedic diet. There are arguments to be made in defense of ghee; it's good for the gut bacteria, and it helps with digestion. But eating a tablespoon of ghee on occasion doesn't mean you do what I used to do and hit the cheese like it's the last edible thing on Earth. Once I dropped sugar, I gave myself permission to eat as much dairy and wheat as I wanted. As long as it wasn't sugar, right? I was eating better; I was thinner, but I was still aging prematurely. Trust me, you don't need that glass of milk, and you really don't need that ice cream after dinner. Dairy is designed, by nature, and now by factories, to be addictive. Gotta get those baby cows to eat it, and gotta get them fat fast.

Give up dairy in all guises—milk, cheese, yogurt, ice cream, ke-fir, butter, cream cheese, and sour cream. Try it for the first 3 weeks of the *Reset* and discover how good it feels to be dairy free.

Why do we even eat dairy? We don't need it. We don't need it from a nutritional standpoint. And, more importantly for those of us good eaters, we don't need from a taste perspective. None of us need dairy to make food tasty. In fact, if you are a lover of Asian cuisines, then you already know this to be true. We don't even need dairy for mouthfeel or umami or whatever else is key when it comes to food. And, dairy is an allergen for most people. If something is an allergen for you then it's inflammatory, and consistent exposure to the allergen leads to chronic inflammation, and then to prema-ture aging.

One of the reasons dairy is bad for us is casein, the protein in cow's milk. Casein has been shown to promote cancer at every stage in the cancer process. Research has also shown that casein is highly addictive. Casein is why we keep craving cheese or whatever creamy food contains dairy. Isn't it telling? The foods that are worst for us are also the most addictive? (It's not like you're going to become a broccoli or apple addict. You may love those foods, but you can't become addicted to them.) "As you digest casein, it breaks apart to release opiates, called *casomorphins*—that is, casein-derived mor-phine-like chemicals. Shortly after you swallow a bite of cheese piz-za these chemicals enter your bloodstream and pass to your brain, and they attach to your opiate receptors. Casomorphins' natural function, presumably, is to provide a bit of feel-good sensation to a nursing calf. And because a calf is weaned very soon, the fat, cholesterol and sodium in milk products are not a problem," says Dr. Neal Barnard, M.D., founder of Physicians Committee for Re-sponsible Medicine.

Casein is also hard for humans to digest; it's why about 75 per-cent of the world's population is allergic to dairy. The other 25 percent, those not allergic, hardly benefit from their consumption of dairy. It can still be a mild allergen, even if it's not an active one, as it is for people like my father and me. The immune system's reactions to casein keep the body in a state of chronic inflammation. That's true for all of us.

Since we humans, like other animals, are not designed to consume the milk from other species, our over-consumption of dairy from cows, goats, and sheep becomes a problem. A big one. I should know, I went through a block (a big one) of swiss or cheddar cheese a week. It was my pre-dinner treat. And I ate organic kefir and goat milk yogurt, thinking it was good for me. But a lot of my digestive and sinus issues were from the supposedly good-for-me, high-in-protein dairy.

And, I'm hardly alone in my intolerance to dairy. "Nearly 50 million Americans have lactose intolerance, a condition in which the body cannot digest significant amounts of a sugar, called lactose, found in milk and other dairy products. The condition occurs when the body is unable to manufacture adequate amounts of lactase, an enzyme needed to break down and digest lactose. If lactose gets through the stomach and small intestines without being digested, it makes its way to the colon, where colonic bacteria ferment it. This results in gas production and excess fluid, causing bloating and diarrhea." From the book *No More Digestive Problems* by Cynthia Yoshida and Deborah Kotz. And, it's likely that more than 50 million Americans are allergic to dairy. But most don't notice their allergy because they're consuming so many other toxins, making it tricky to discern which foods are causing them inflammatory issues.

I recommend dropping dairy because it's aging. And, for most people consumption of dairy hampers the digestion and absorption of nutrients. Consumption of dairy leads to skin problems, and there have even been studies showing that it contributes to cellulite. Most of us are lactose-intolerant, never realizing our weight gain, eczema, acne, and other skin rashes are caused by dairy in our diet.

If dairy was inflammatory before, now it is downright poisonous. Consider how cows live nowadays. They are genetically manipulated, given antibiotics and hormones so that their milk yield increases, and their living environments are atrocious. Milk is contaminated with cow's blood, pus, pesticides, and hormones. You ingest what they are fed and the toxins in the environment flow from their milk to you. Dairy is a dirty food. It's one of the top foods recalled most often due to serious contamination.

And, if we want to lose weight or stay lean, guess what, dairy makes us fat. It was designed to fatten the calf in a short amount of time, and that's what it does to us. Dairy can make you very sick too; it is loaded with estrogen. Here's something that is kind of obvious once you think about it: cow's milk has estrogen metabolites because it comes from lactating cows. "Most breast cancers are estrogen receptor positive, so elevated blood levels of estrogen increase the risk of breast cancer. Cow's milk is designed to help a calf grow to several hundred pounds within a short period of time, so cow's milk increases production of a hormone called insulin-like growth factor, or IGF-1, which helps to fuel this growth. But dairy products also increase IGF-1 levels in humans; the dairy industries own studies show this. The problem is that IGF-1 is a powerful cancer promoter in humans; there are clear links between IGF-1 levels and breast, lung, colon, and prostate cancers. In fact, the link between low-fat cow's milk and prostate cancer is stronger than the link between smoking and lung cancer." Pamela Popper, Ph.D., ND, explains in the book *Food Over Medicine*.

It's hard for me to find the upside to eating dairy. The protein you get from it is harder for the body to use as fuel than a plant-based one like tofu. Dairy proteins have been linked to so many inflammatory and autoimmune issues and diseases, like obesity, asthma, allergies, chronic constipation, chronic ear infections in children, multiple sclerosis, autoimmune diseases, breast cancer (as Dr. Popper explained), type 1 diabetes, and osteoporosis, that it seems good, common sense to drop it from any diet. Dairy, like meat, is acidic; it leaches calcium out of the body. The pleasure you get from a bite of cheesecake or a trip around a cheese plate isn't worth the pain that comes later.

Another scary thing about the most prevalent type of dairy in America, cow's milk, is that it contains viruses that promote cancer, especially leukemia and lymphoma. In nations where dairy is most consumed disease follows, especially leukemia and lymphoma. Imaging feeding a child a big cold glass of milk, a.k.a bovine leukemia virus (BLV); 89 percent of herds of cattle in the United States are infected with bovine leukemia. We ingest this virus when we consume dairy. While studies are not totally conclusive that humans infected with BLV contract leukemia, it does seem we may be at risk. In a recent study, scientists found, "BLV in human tissues indicates a risk for the acquisition and proliferation of this virus in humans."

Quit dairy or, at the very least, limit your consumption. And, for those first 3 weeks of the *Reset*, give it up. *It's an Ageless Rule.*

If you worry you'll miss dairy, especially cheese, I get it. I did too. But, there are so many amazing alternatives to dairy. I was surprised giving it up wasn't an issue for me, and I'm a big dairy queen. If you crave that creamy, rich mouthfeel and taste, try coconut milk, tofu, tahini-based sauces or aiolis made with egg and olive oil. You don't need dairy to enjoy flavorful food. Just ask any good vegan cook. And if you really love cheese and sour cream, you'll be happy to learn on this diet/lifestyle, there are all kinds of foods you can make and eat that answer the craving for something rich and creamy. Homemade hummus with tahini hits that sweet spot. So does avocado in guacamole. Or avocado whisked in with a bright vinaigrette. I love creamy, smoky baba ghanouj. And then, there's cashew spread, better than sour cream on black beans, tofu, or on a burrito bowl with grass-fed beef. And what about vegan green goddess dressing and black bean dip? So delicious, I'll eat it standing in my kitchen, over the bowl with a pile of carrots. There are so many options and so many great recipes that taste as good or better than a big hunk of inflammatory cheese and dollop of addicting sour cream. If you need something creamy in your coffee try a plant based milk (coconut, cashew, almond, or hemp milk), all very easy to make at home.

Now that I've done my fair share of fear mongering, here's good news. Kale, collards, broccoli, and spinach have plenty of bioavailable calcium and protein. Kale smoothie > milk, all day long.

CHAPTER 15

DROP WHEAT (THE 3ᴿᴰ INFLAMMATORY FOOD)

Don't be so refined . . .
Eat more whole grains, less white flour.

Wheat is the third and last food we quit while on the *Reset*, at least for the first 28 days. Why drop wheat? Because it's often inflammatory, and inflammation ages you. Drop it for the first 4 weeks on the *Reset* to give yourself a clean slate and help you understand if wheat triggers inflammation in you.

Notice I wrote drop wheat, not gluten. Though the first 4 weeks of the *Reset* is gluten-free, it's not because gluten is necessarily inflammatory. It's to give you a chance to learn what is an allergen for you. And, I'm not going to tell you gluten is the villain in this chapter, because I don't know. Nobody knows yet why so many claim to be allergic to gluten. Without the scientific evidence I can't say for sure why there is an uptick in allergies to gluten. But I do believe our intolerance to wheat and gluten must be related in part to the health of the microbiome. A healthy gut with plenty of beneficial bacteria makes digestion of potentially inflammatory grains, including wheat, much easier. And, one of the goals of Ageless Diet is to improve the overall health of your gut. Meanwhile, though, for the first 4 weeks of the *Reset* drop wheat and gluten from your diet. Because, bottom-line, modern wheat is inflammatory, and the goal here is to cool down all diet and lifestyle related inflammation.

I love bread. And bread made from intact ancient grains (spelt, teff, and heirloom wheat like Kamut and Einkorn), allowed to naturally ferment or long-ferment, is something most of us could easily digest. It can be high in fiber and nutrients. However, most bread we eat is from refined, highly processed wheat. Here are some of the chemicals added to processed modern wheat: *ammonium chloride, azodicarbonamide, benzoyl peroxide (in acne creams), calcium propionate, chlorine dioxide (chlorine!), dextrose, diacetyl tartaric acid, esters of mono and diglycerides, vital wheat gluten* (added, extra gluten that is virtually indestructible*), potassium bromate, sodium stearoyl 2 lactylate, starch enzymes.* This isn't ageless food. This bread from modern dwarf wheat, with all these additives including vital wheat gluten, is bad. Because while gluten may not be the enemy, you don't need extra gluten added to your bread. You don't need any additives in any of your foods.

And modern wheat is everywhere, hiding in most processed foods and in thousands of other products, including cosmetics. Wheat is versatile, making it the perfect hidden ingredient in so many things: soups, sauces, gravies, dressings, spreads, snack foods, processed meats, frozen vegetables, etc. It's also addictive. Ever hear the word gluteomorphin? I can go months without it, but the minute I've sampled a roll in a nice Manhattan restaurant that basket of bread is mine, all mine. As my father Tom would say, all food bets are off. I'm back on bread. At first, I feel fine, but after a week of steady sandwich and bagel eating, my digestion is wonky, and I'm losing energy. It's sometimes a subtle thing, but I feel the ill effects from wheat sooner or later, usually sooner. For Scott, it's almost immediate. Digestion issues, asthma attacks, sinus headaches, aches and pains . . . the popping of ibuprofen begins. And we're not even allergic to gluten! We can eat other whole grains containing gluten with no problem. In fact, we love whole, intact grains.

But we're not talking about dropping intact grains from our diet. We're talking about conventional wheat with all this nasty stuff added to process it. It seems logical to assume we weren't designed to handle the many toxic chemicals used in producing wheat. Did you know pesticides are routinely employed in wheat production? So, maybe the culprit isn't gluten, per se, but instead some super-charged Frankenstein wheat that destroys the farmland and our bodies.

Modern dwarf wheat was introduced around 1960. It was developed via crossbreeding and genetic manipulation, thus changing the nutrient and protein composition of the plant. This wheat has significantly less of the important minerals like magnesium, iron, zinc and copper than heritage wheat. With its short stalks and roots, it produces big kernels that are easily harvested by machine. This means they can farm a higher density of plants within limited acreage. And, it's this density or overpopulation that allows plant and soil disease flourish, thus requiring more pesticides. Modern short-stalk or dwarf wheat also needs extreme amounts of water. So much water that acreage dedicated to this crop dries up non-replenishing aquifers. Especially dire as water becomes more and more scarce around the world, and when water is pumped onto the soil year after year, residual minerals in the irrigation water concentrate and non-saline soil becomes saline, leading to toxic farmland. Modern wheat requires chemical fertilizers—and lots of them—because nature can't provide enough nutrients in the soil to the meet the plants' demands in order to flourish. The various petro-chemical fertilizers, pesticides, herbicides, and fungicides required in modern wheat horticulture are way too many for the health of the consumers and the land.

And this dwarf wheat, with none of the nutrients of heritage wheat and too many toxins to contemplate, is everywhere. It's in almost everything, processed foods, soups, sauces, and of course breads. It's a huge part of the western diet. This wheat is an addictive appetite stimulant. The proteins in wheat are converted to polypeptides called exorphins. Like the endorphins we get naturally from exercise, they bind to the opioid receptors in the brain. This makes you high and addicted, similar to a heroin addict. The wheat polypeptides get into your bloodstream and cross the blood brain barrier. Guess what they're called? Gluteomorphins. Gluten morphine. Now I know why I kept eating bread long after I was full. I've never done that with vegetables, because they are not addictive. Binge eaters never overdose on black-eyed peas and collards; they binge on junk food. Because junk food is often loaded with added wheat, sugars, fats, and salt. Modern wheat is made up of a super starch, called amylopectin, which is fattening. *It's designed to make you fat.* Two slices of refined (and processed) whole wheat bread spike your blood sugar more than 2 tablespoons of table sugar.

There is mounting evidence that modern wheat is much more harmful to those with celiac disease and people with gluten sensitivity, compared to older, heirloom breeds like Emmer, Einkorn, and Kamut wheat.

In fact, I had no issues with wheat as a child. We ate freshly baked bread all the time. It was a staple. We also ate whole grains containing gluten: farro, barley, spelt, rye, bulgur wheat, and oats. But, I think, because we bought all our food at the local co-op, the local health food store, it was not highly processed stuff. The wheat was from small farms, farms that didn't spray their crops with pesticides. (Remember how pesticides, sometimes used in farming wheat, disrupt the functioning of beneficial bacteria in your gut, destroying the microbiome and leading to all sorts of issues, digestive, autoimmune, and otherwise?) The wheat my dad used in baking bread was always organic heritage wheat. It had a nubby texture and a nutty fragrance; it wasn't super fine like flours we buy now at the grocery store. Our bread was made with whole grains and water, allowed to rise slowly, naturally. It's really wondrous to me that all you need for a really great loaf of bread is whole grain, water, and plenty of time for it to ferment. But after the age of 8, once my parents separated, we started eating what other people ate, bags of squashy refined whole wheat bread, milk, grape jellies, sweetened peanut butter, and so much sugar, and my headaches started.

It's the wheat we have an issue with, not necessarily gluten. And, though a gluten-free diet is all the rage these days, people are still overweight and inflamed. And, ironically, most people claiming gluten intolerance don't even know what gluten is. The gluten-free industry is now a billion dollar one, and a lot of folks think if they steer clear of gluten, they can eat whatever they want. But it's the processed foods, dairy, modern wheat, and sugar that make people suffer from inflammation overload. And though most of us are aware of the dangers of gluten for a few people, especially the 1 percent with celiac disease, we often don't know why gluten makes them sick or why we should avoid it. We just believe that gluten is bad and it makes us sick. But the issue is more complex. It involves inflammatory foods, a gut imbalance, and general poor health.

Gluten is the sticky protein that makes bread rise. Actually, gluten is not a single protein, but a family of different proteins. If you're a baker, like me, you've probably used plenty of high-gluten flour to create loftier pastries made from more pliable dough. This is what gluten does, and dwarf wheat is designed to be much higher in gluten proteins than our old, Biblical wheat—that staff of life stuff. More scientifically engineered gluten with more additives for processing wheat seems to equal more inflammation and allergic response. And, it could lead to a damaged gut.

To give us an opportunity to discover what is, in fact, an allergen we drop both wheat and gluten from our diet for the first 28 days of the *Reset*. Then you will know if you're actually gluten-intolerant. Or perhaps, it's the modern wheat you have an issue with. Most of us probably have no allergy to gluten, but rather an intolerance to products made from modern dwarf wheat. Scientists researching gluten allergies are now saying that non-celiac gluten sensitivity is a misnomer, and we should call any sensitivity wheat intolerance. However, if you decided wheat and/or gluten is an allergen, drop it immediately. There are so many whole grains you can eat: grains and pseudocereals that taste really good, nourish you, fill you up, and keep you healthy.

For me, modern wheat in processed breads and pastries and dough is inflammatory, so I dropped it from my diet. And, you may discover the same thing to be true for you. After 4 weeks reintroduce whole grains containing gluten, and you can decide whether they make you feel good or bad. If you experience bloating, congestion, any digestive issues, or you feel sick, tired, and achy, drop wheat for good.

If, after the first 28 days on the Ageless Diet, you find that wheat—whole, organic wheat—and other whole grains with gluten are not allergens for you, enjoy them as part of a balanced diet. Make sure, though, you're eating the purest, organic whole grains you can find. If you want bread, we recommend sticking with sprouted-grain or long-fermented bread. My favorite is a wild yeast, long-ferment sourdough bread. You can also delve into bread baking, a wonderfully rewarding process, with an irresistible result. Try it old school, find a whole grain you like the looks of, add filtered water, salt, and then give it enough time to naturally ferment. If gluten isn't an issue for you, enjoy steel-cut oats and other whole grains like freekeh, wheat berries, bulgur wheat, barley, farro, and rye. Continue to avoid regular breads, pastries, doughnuts, croissants, muffins, pizza dough, cookies, bagels, and packaged cereals. And stay away from gluten-free breads, pastas, and pastries. They're typically high in sugar and about as bad as eating a loaf of regular white bread dusted with sugar. When it comes to reintroducing whole wheat and other whole grains with gluten, or grains like oats that are tricky for those with gluten sensitivity, do it the week following the reintroduction of dairy. You don't want to conflate your allergic reactions or non-reactions. And then observe, *feel,* how your brain and body react to wheat and gluten.

I'm not eating pizza or any other of those breads, muffins, bagels, and pastries I used to love. I don't have celiac disease, and I'm not gluten intolerant. But I feel better limiting wheat in my diet, and limiting the gluten I consume to certain whole, intact grains. Scott feels much better without modern wheat in his diet. He has more energy, fewer allergy attacks, and less aches and pains. The other good thing about dropping wheat is that we end up eating more vegetables, experimenting with naturally gluten-free cuisines from around the world, trying new ingredients, and sampling different whole grains. In short, limiting wheat (and dairy) in our diet created an opportunity for Scott and me. We eat a much more varied diet with fresh vegetables. And that's a win/win.

CHAPTER 16

THERE'S ALWAYS HOPE

"You can set yourself up to be sick,
or you can choose to stay well."
—WAYNE DYER

Despairing over all the sugar, wheat, dairy, and junk foods you've eaten? Don't be. First of all, you can't have consumed more crap food than me. It's impossible. I was the number one sugar fiend, dairy queen, breadbasket lover—the top fast food customer. And secondly, there's always hope. You can almost always reverse the damage done. Don't freak out if you're looking at decades of over consumption of processed foods and sugar, wondering what's the point of trying to change. You can reduce inflammation. You can feel better. You can lose weight. None of you have eaten more fast food meals, more sweets, candy, and desserts than I have. If I can drop sugar and junk foods, you can. It is possible to heal the body through diet and lifestyle and reverse the negative effects. You can stop chronic inflammation and premature aging. You can turn back the clock. It's never too late to change.

Good food and a positive lifestyle work miracles. My 50-something friend Blair looks about 36 these days. He's lean, strong, happier, and younger looking. Lines have smoothed out, the bloom is back on the rose. When I first met Blair about 28 months ago, he was tired, haggard looking, and puffy. He had some extra weight, and his face looked jowly, his eyes sad. He wasn't sleeping well. I'm one of those annoying people, when I learn something that works I want to shout it from a mountaintop. Blair was a willing participant, because he felt so bad, and he knew he could feel better.

Within 3 weeks, the inflammation had gone down, he was sleeping better, and exercising daily. His libido was up, and his energy was high. He felt good and he looked great. Twelve months later, the years kept falling away. Twenty-five-year-old men wanted to go out with him, and he had the best summer of his life this year. "The Ageless Diet transformed me. This lifestyle works. Even better, it makes for more easeful living. I'm in my 50's and I regularly get mistaken for a man much younger. I feel and look lighter, stronger, and younger. I love food. I've learned how to cook healthier, and my friends enjoy my cooking so much they prefer when I am the dinner party host. Life is fun again. I'm living a sustainable lifestyle, better for me and the planet. And I look great while doing it." It's not always easy; the Ageless Diet is work. But it's work that will save your life. When your diet/lifestyle is inflammatory you're prone to depression, sleeplessness, and fatigue. It's not just your body you're affecting.

"A growing body of evidence links particular foods and eating patterns with lower levels of inflammatory biomarkers. Both epidemiological (skin) studies and intervention trials support a link between diet and a reduced risk of many chronic diseases, and experts believe that the diet-inflammation connection might be one explanation. In a 2006 study published in the Journal of the American College of Cardiology, scientists found that diets high in refined starches, sugars, saturated fats, and trans fats and low in fruits, vegetables, whole grains, and omega-3 fatty acids appear to turn on the inflammatory response. But a diet rich in whole foods, including healthful carbohydrates and fat and protein sources, along with regular exercise and not smoking, seems to cool down inflammation." (From *Today's Dietitian*)

Most people are prematurely aging; they are sick and dying from the typical American lifestyle. Years of alcohol and drugs (both pharmaceutical and recreational), too many processed foods, dehydration (over-consumption of flavored waters, sodas, coffees), almost no of physical exercise, and many hours spent looking at TV and computer screens have given people:

- Significantly weakened eyes
- Wrinkles by age 30 or even earlier
- Brain damage, depression, addiction, ADD, ADHD, irritability, and nervousness
- A body that is weak, stiff, and lacking in energy
- A severely diminished, less vibrant mind and body

It doesn't have to be this way; you don't have age conventionally. You don't have to buy what (food, drugs, toxins) they're selling. You can make simple, easy choices that turn it all around. Your body is an integrated part of an information and energy system. There is no separation with how your body feels, your gut, and your brain—all is connected. You can feel better NOW.

CHAPTER 17

SAVE YOUR LIFE, SAVE THE WORLD: FALL IN LOVE WITH REAL FOOD

"Don't eat anything your great grandmother wouldn't recognize as food. When you pick up that box of portable yogurt tubes, or eat something with 15 ingredients you can't pronounce, ask yourself, 'What are those things doing there?'"
—MICHAEL POLLAN

Anyone born after 1960 has grown up in a corporate sponsored nutritional fantasyland, full of fake food advertised as healthy. I know it's an uphill battle. There's a trillion-plus-dollar machine in place to keep us buying and consuming food-like substances. But you don't have to wage war on the machine to win. All you need to do is feed yourself REAL FOOD.

Here is an easy basic rule to shop by: If it's got a label, and the label doesn't read something simple like black beans, water, salt, then it's not exactly food; it's something constructed in a lab, not a kitchen. Eat foods that come without labels, foods that grow in nature. Or as Michael Pollan succinctly puts it: "If it came from a plant, eat it. If it was made in a plant, don't." You shouldn't need to whip out your phone and do a Google search for every ingredient on a label. Processed foods are hard to avoid, I know. They're everywhere, and a lot of them are considered healthy. But 98 percent aren't. These foods will inflame you and age you. They also do a number on the planet. So take the time when you shop to seek out real, whole foods. Make your own snacks, cook most of your own meals, avoid packaged foods, most of which are processed like the plague—a plague of inflammation, disease, obesity, and premature aging.

Given his work, Peter Lehner, executive director of the Natural Resources Defense Council, is hyper aware of the real story behind processed foods and their engineered addictiveness. The food industry spends trillions convincing us to consume what they're selling, at great cost to our health. Most of these additives deemed "safe" for consumption are in fact the opposite; they are quite dangerous.

Mr. Lehner writes in an article for *Live Science*: "When we pick up a package of food at the store—cereal, frozen pizza, chips, an energy drink, a nutrition bar, cake—we assume that everything in it is OK to eat. Companies wouldn't be allowed sell those foods otherwise, right? But because of a giant loophole in food safety law—the 'generally recognized as safe,' or GRAS, loophole—chemical manufacturers can decide for themselves if the product they've created is safe to consume. Their safety assessments don't have to be reviewed or approved by anyone else, and often manufacturers don't even have to disclose the name of the additive, or how it's used, to the FDA or to the public. Often, the agency isn't even notified when chemical additives enter our food supply."

Obviously, given that these are profit-driven companies, these foods are designed to encourage *overconsumption:* "The widespread use of chemical additives is just one of several deep-rooted problems in our industrialized food system. Our food system encourages the consumption of processed and packaged foods over fresh, healthier, locally grown foods. We end up craving the sugar that sneaks into processed foods, and so we keep buying more of it— and we assume that it's safe to eat," explains Mr. Lehner. Because there are few to no limits on what manufacturers can put into processed foods, "some additives which manufacturers claimed to be 'generally recognized as safe' had been linked to fetal leukemia in human cell tests, or testicular degeneration in animal tests, or, according to FDA scientists, may trigger an allergic reaction in people with peanut allergies." The impact of our current food system on our bodies and the planet is hard to overstate. The consumption of processed foods, the industrial farming, and the sheer amount of food wasted—almost 40 percent of food is uneaten and tossed in the trash—results in chronic inflammation and pollution, in our bodies and, "throughout the natural systems that sustain our health and the planet," Mr. Lehner points out.

Do yourself a huge favor and stop buying all processed foods. Your wallet will thank you too. A package of "healthy" low-fat snacks is much more expensive than a bag of organic apples. It's 100 percent more affordable to eat healthy, real, whole foods (even organic) than spend money on seemingly cheap junk food.

From renowned cookbook writer Mark Bittman *of The New York Times*: "In general, despite extensive government subsidies, hyperprocessed food remains more expensive than food cooked at home. You can serve a roasted chicken with vegetables along with a simple salad and milk for about $14, and feed four or even six people. If that's too much money, substitute a meal of rice and canned beans with bacon, green peppers and onions; it's easily enough for four people and costs about $9." It's also more affordable in the long run. You won't get sick or fat; you won't need expensive drugs to fight inflammatory diseases or serious medical attention at your doctor's office and hospital.

Don't eat junk foods and you won't get addicted, and if you do eat it, stop right now. Treat yourself to a real meal with real food. Get cooking. You have the time; we all do. Study after study shows that almost all of us, regardless of income level, watch at least two and a half hours of TV a day, and often it's more like four hours. We have the time to cook. It connects us to what we eat in a way that enhances our enjoyment of the food.

Plus, that junk food is fully loaded with super sugars, super starches, and super additives that lead to super weight gain. From

Mr. Bittman's article: "The engineering behind hyperprocessed food makes it virtually addictive. A 2009 study by the Scripps Research Institute indicates that overconsumption of fast food 'triggers addiction-like neuroaddictive responses' in the brain, making it harder to trigger the release of dopamine. In other words the more fast food we eat, the more we need to give us pleasure; thus the report suggests that the same mechanisms underlie drug addiction and obesity." I know this firsthand. After 2 days of double cheeseburgers, fries, and a diet cola at my favorite fast food place, I wanted it every day. In fact, I couldn't stay away even if I wanted to, my addiction was too intense.

It behooves the makers of these processed foods to promote the argument that the obesity epidemic is the result of a failure in personal responsibility. But that's a lie, and it's unfair. It places all the blame on the individual. The real truth is scarier. What they're selling, what we're buying, is as addictive as serious, outlawed hard drugs.

Processed foods are even sold at your local natural food store. We're told all the time that going vegan is really good for our health. Yes, it can be, but vegan prepared foods, snacks, frozen dinners, chips, cookies, faux cheese and meat, sauces, fruit and nut bars, desserts—you know the food I'm talking about—are just as bad as Twinkies. If you're vegan, skip the vegan cookies and Tofurkey, and keep it simple, stick with vegetables, fruits, legumes, nuts, seeds, tofu, whole grains, and good plant-based fats.

When you eat badly, to comfort yourself because you're having a tough day, you actually make your day worse. Again, this I know from personal experience. Feeding a craving feels good while I'm doing it, but then within a half hour I feel worse than before, emotionally and physically. That Happy Meal just isn't worth the brief high, and it doesn't make me very happy. Don't punish yourself with crap food. The good news is eating ageless can lift your mood, make a bad day better, *and make a good day amazing*. You handle the inevitable stresses of life with greater ease when you take care of your body.

What you eat, and how you live, can reduce your risk for cancers growing and spreading. Diet and exercise, not to mention sleep and meditation, have been shown to reduce recurrences of cancer and extend survival. But the best way to treat cancer is through prevention. Diets high in sugar and trans and saturated fats make people obese, and, as some doctors say, obesity is a bona fide tumor promoter. The same diet/lifestyle that makes us obese creates a chronic inflammatory state. And, a chronic inflammatory state makes it easy for cancers to grow and spread throughout the body.

Manufactured fats, found in processed food-like substances, in fast foods, margarine, and highly processed carbohydrates and oils, age us in part because they clog arteries. This clogging takes away elasticity from skin because water can't get through. But, happily, almost all natural plant-based fats are good. Natural monounsaturated fats, those in cold-pressed organic oils— olive oil, coconut oil, hemp oil, avocado oil, and sesame oil—are rich in vitamin E. This "helps stabilize cellular walls and protect against oxidation and free radicals that age skin," says registered dietitian Jen Brewer, author of *Stop Dieting and Start Losing Weight*.

As with fat, not all carbohydrates (carbs) are bad. In fact, we need carbohydrates and starches. What we don't need is hyper-processed carbs. Highly processed, refined carbohydrates (simple carbs) are bad. But, plant foods are full of healthy carbohydrates; these include fruits, vegetables, legumes, seeds, and whole (intact) grains. Grains are of two types: true cereals (grasses) and pseudocereals (nongrasses). Eating a diet rich in healthy carbs, lean proteins, and good fats can reverse the damage a diet high in sugar, simple carbs, and processed foods has done. It's never too late to reverse damage and turn back the clock. It's not just cancer and heart disease that respond to a mostly plant-based diet. This type of anti-inflammatory diet helps protect against premature aging, obesity, depression, dementia, diabetes, autoimmune diseases, and bone, kidney, eye, and brain diseases.

I'm living proof that an Ageless Diet works, as are Scott, Katrien, Lee-Ann, Chris, Blair, Anna, and an ever-increasing number of others. We're all healthier and fitter than we've ever been in our adult lives. We're reverse aging. And, it wasn't hard to do.

Ok, sugar, dairy, wheat, and processed foods are out. So, what can you eat? The list of ageless-approved foods is so long, I put it in the back of the book for an easy reference.

By eating ageless you are saving yourself and the world around you. You can change your life, you can reverse the premature aging, and you can contribute to making the planet a healthier place. It starts with you; it ends with you. Alice Waters puts it this way: "Eating is a political act, but in the way the ancient Greeks used the word 'political'—not just to mean having to do with voting in an election, but to mean 'of, or pertaining to, all our interactions with other people'—from the family to the school, to the neighborhood, the nation, and the world. Every single choice we make about food matters, at every level. The right choice saves the world."

CHAPTER 18

EAT LESS MEAT.
EAT BETTER MEAT.

*"A high-protein diet—particularly if
the proteins are derived from animals—is nearly
as bad as smoking for your health."*
—Professor Valter Longo,
University of Southern California.

For the good of our own health and our planet's wellbeing, it's time we restored meat to its status as a luxury—delicious, expensive, and rare. The last time we ate this way, before the post-World War II boom, hips were bigger than waists. Nowadays meat is cheap and readily available and waistlines have disappeared, as people get fatter and sicker.

Most people eat too much meat. Everyone I know at the gym is obsessed with protein. They believe high protein consumption builds lean muscles and a thin body. *Lose the protein myth.* Thanks to all these meat heavy diets popular now, protein is king. You don't need to eat a pound of beef every day to look like an Olympic champion. Thanks to a very powerful meat industry, billions spent on advertising and bad intel, most of us have been tricked into thinking more steak means a healthier, thinner, stronger body. But plant-based eaters get their quota of protein met easily, thanks to grains, seeds, legumes, and vegetables naturally high in protein without any of the inflammatory side effects. There are powerful herbivores in the animal kingdom, rhinos, hippos, elephants, and bulls to name a few, who thrive on plants. And we can too. I'm not promoting a vegan diet, though eating mostly vegan is smart, nor am I saying all meat is bad. After all, I'm an omnivore. I'm simply saying that plants can be excellent and very tasty sources of protein.

Don't be misled by incorrect information. You do need protein in every meal, but you only need about 0.36 grams of protein for each pound of body weight. The sweet spot for protein consumption is 40-60 grams per day. And, no more than 20 percent of the daily calories in your diet should be protein. In fact, it's recommended that 10-15 percent of our daily calories come from protein (about 56 grams for men and 46 for women). The exact amount of protein you need depends largely on your body weight, but it's roughly 1 gram for every 2.2 pounds. Nutritionists advise aiming for at least 12 grams of protein per meal and 5-7 grams per snack. The average American man consumes about 102 grams of protein a day, and the average woman eats about 70 grams of protein a day. We love protein and almost everyone we know is aging too quickly.

Excessive consumption of animal protein is aging. A study from Cleveland Clinic's Wellness Institute shows eating red meat more than once a week is linked to skin wrinkling, as well as serious health risks. According to the research, the high level of carnitine, a compound abundant in animal protein, can harden blood vessel walls, causing skin to crease prematurely.

If you still think that a high-protein diet is the way to go, consider how much animal protein the average American consumes, and then consider this fact: of 22 industrialized countries, the U.S. has the highest obesity statistics. The average American consumes an excessive amount of meat and dairy. Two thirds of Americans over age 20 are overweight, and nearly one third of Americans over age 20 are obese; excessive consumption of animal-based proteins often leads to obesity.

Eric Schlosser, in his book *Fast Food Nation,* pointed out that the annual health care costs in the United States stemming from obesity approaches **$240 billion**. That's a huge amount of money wasted on a totally preventable issue. What if we simply changed our diet and lifestyle? It's easy enough to do, and unlike going to the doctor, a few, simple changes in your lifestyle won't cost you an arm and a leg.

Though you may not need a big hunk of meat every day, obviously, you do need to eat protein with every meal and in any snacks. This requirement could be met with a few Brazil nuts and almonds. But up to and beyond 30 percent of your daily calories from protein a day is aging and inflammatory.

There have been many studies of late pointing out that people who consume excessive protein, especially animal-based proteins, are at a much greater risk for cancer and other inflammatory diseases than those who consume a moderate amount of protein. A recent study found that "cheese can be just as bad for you as smoking. It all boiled down to the protein in cheese and the source it came from—animals. The study showed that middle-aged individuals consuming an animal-based high protein diet were almost twice more likely to die early and four times more likely to die of cancer, not to mention significantly more likely to age prematurely. Moderate protein intake, however, was found to be beneficial after the age of 65 due to a decrease in the growth hormone IGF-I. The same correlations were found in smokers. Interesting that smoking cigarettes and over-consumption of animal-based protein has similar effects on the body in terms of disease promoting and premature aging. In the study, researchers defined a 'high-protein' diet as deriving at least 20 percent of calories from protein, including both plant-based and animal-based protein. A 'moderate' protein diet includes 10 to 19 percent of calories from protein, and a 'low-protein' diet includes less than 10 percent protein," writes Kristin Kirkpatrick, MS, RD, LD, manager of Wellness Nutrition Services at the Cleveland Clinic Wellness Institute, in *U.S. News & World Report*.

A person on a typical high-protein diet consumes 38 percent of his daily calories from protein. That's a lot of protein. Research from a study published in *Cell Metabolism Journal* suggests that, despite the popularity in high protein diets like Atkins and Paleo, it would be wise to eat the opposite way, because a protein-rich diet increases risk of cancer. Protein from animal sources—meat and dairy—is the source of the risk; plant-based proteins are much safer. Those who consumed high-to-moderate amounts of animal protein had a three times higher chance of dying of cancer. But these risks and inflammation disappeared among participants whose high-protein diet was mainly plant-based. Experiments on cells show the amino acids that proteins are made of reduces cellular protection and increases damage to DNA, pointing to a fact that excessive protein consumption could be aging.

So, what happens to the excess protein consumed? Dr. Popper, Executive Director of the Wellness Forum, explains the process in the book *Food Over Medicine*: "If you consume too much protein, even plant protein, you simply have to get rid of the excess; we can't store much protein [in our bodies]. What the body will do is convert some of the surplus protein to carbohydrate because that's readily usable for energy. In the process of doing this, the body has to get rid of nitrogen from the amino acid chains, as carbohydrate does not include nitrogen. As the body releases nitrogen from the amino acid chains, the nitrogen throws off a lot of toxic by-products like urea and ammonia, which are detoxified by the kidneys and liver, causing a lot of stress on those organs. Alzheimer's is rarely present in the plant-eating populations. It's a disease of the western diet. It's a vascular disease that is most prevalent in the populations, like ours, that eat the most meat. Rheumatoid arthritis is almost always diet and lifestyle related, and is particularly related to the consumption of animal foods."

If you eat an anti-inflammatory diet, full of good fats, nuts, seeds, whole grains, vegetables, legumes and fruits, and free of processed foods, sugar, dairy, and wheat, you will naturally get an adequate amount of protein. After that, any excess protein will ultimately be stored as fat. In general, excess calories, regardless of the source, whether they're calories from protein or not, are stored by the body as fat. Once your daily protein needs are met, your body has two options for dealing with any excess protein in your diet. If your calorie intake is low that day your cells convert excess amino acids to molecules that can burn as fuel. If however, you consume enough calories throughout the day your body has no choice but to convert the extra protein to fatty acids and store them in your adipose tissue, a.k.a. fat. Meaning you're storing excess fat in your body for a rainy day, which would be fine in the Paleolithic era, when you were never sure if your next meal was around the corner, across the savanna, and over the river. Storing fat was great from a feast or famine point of view. But we live in a totally different world, and excess fat is not what most of us need. Plus, those Paleolithic ancestors of ours were lucky to live to 40. Is that your goal? Or are you hoping to live to a vibrant 90 and beyond? If so, limit your consumption of protein.

Concerned about getting enough protein from plants? Don't be. You would be amazed at the grams of protein in vegetables, legumes, soy, eggs, grains, seeds, and nuts. Oftentimes a salad really is all you need.

Here are some examples of how much protein certain foods contain:

- 1 cup cooked broccoli = 4 grams of protein

- 2 tablespoons of almonds = 4 grams of protein

- 1 cup of brown rice = 5 grams of protein

- 1 egg = 6 grams of protein

- 1 ounce steak = 7 grams of protein

- 1 cup of quinoa = 8 grams of protein

- 5 ounces of tofu = 12 grams of protein

- 1 cup of lentils = 18 grams of protein

For maximum agelessness most of us need to eat more good carbohydrates. What are good carbs? Plants. And they have many of the same essential amino acids (proteins) as meat. Your body breaks up all protein sources into amino acids. Plus, vegetables like broccoli, spinach and kale have more protein, calcium, iron, and fiber per calorie than beef! One hundred calories of broccoli has about 11 grams of protein. In a steak, one hundred calories equals 6-8 grams of protein, depending on the cut of beef. A vegetable like kale is also high in omega-3 and omega-6 fatty acids. Bonus, kale is an anti-inflammatory. Plant-based proteins don't have any saturated fat, and they are usually lower in calories.

While on the *Reset,* I recommend limiting your meat consumption (and making sure to eat only 100 percent grass-fed, pasture-raised beef, bison, lamb, rabbit, pig, goose, ostrich, chicken, quail, turkey, guinea fowl, duck, partridge, squab, and so on) to no more than three times a week. Once or twice a week would be ideal.

Why grass-fed? One, because it is higher in omega-3 fatty acids than regular, grain-fed or grain-finished beef. Two, it is rich in conjugated linoleic acid, beta-carotene, iron, zinc and B vitamins. (Linoleic acid is a polyunsaturated fatty acid. It is one of two fatty acids that we can't produce ourselves and must get from food. Linoleic acid is used by the body to make other types of omega-6 fatty acids. Some linoleic fat is essential, but most of us are getting way too much from processed foods and vegetable oils like safflower. Get your linoleic acid from nuts and seeds and, occasionally, grass-fed beef.) Three, grass-fed beef has less saturated fat than the grain-fed counterpart. Four, grass-fed cattle are healthier, which means healthier beef. Pasture grazing is in keeping with their natural lifestyle and diet. They are less likely to be infected with disease and less likely to pass that disease or infection on to you. Industrial farming does nobody any favors, not the animals, not the plants, not the environment. If you can bypass big agriculture, factory farming, and industrial beef production, do it. Your body and your planet will thank you.

As Jo Robinson, author of *Eating on the Wild Side,* puts it on her website, EatWild.com: "When you choose to eat meat, eggs, and dairy products from animals raised on pasture, you are improving the welfare of the animals, helping to put an end to environmental degradation, helping small-scale ranchers and farmers make a living from the land, helping to sustain rural communities, and giving your family the healthiest possible food. It's a win-win-win-win situation."

And, it's relatively easy to find grass-fed meat these days. Most grocery and health food stores carry grass-fed beef, pasture-raised eggs, free-range chicken and turkey. Check EatWild.com for more information about where to find and buy grass-fed beef, and for more information about pasture-raised farming.

Curbing our consumption of meat is healthier, and it can have significant environmental impact too. Animal agriculture accounts for a full 19 percent of greenhouse gases—that's more than the transportation sector. Part of looking and feeling ageless is taking care of the world around us. It's hard to feel ageless if you're living in a toxic waste dump, right?

Mark Bittman writes that eating as much meat as we do is "damaging to our health and the environment for a variety of reasons, including rampant antibiotic use; the devotion of more than a third of our global cropland to feeding animals; and the resulting degradation of the environment from that crop and its unimaginable overuse of chemicals, soil and water. Even if large quantities of industrially produced animal products were safe to eat, the environmental costs are demonstrable and huge. And so the argument 'eat less meat but eat better meat' makes sense from every perspective. If you raise fewer animals, you can treat them more humanely and reduce their environmental impact."

If we want to be ageless it's time for all of us to **"eat less meat but eat better meat."**

And if you want to go vegan or vegetarian and skip the grass-fed beef you easily can. It's not only beef that is full of iron and other nutrients. Vegetables are high in iron, beta-carotene, zinc, and B vitamins, among many other vital nutrients. One cup of broccoli is full of calcium, manganese, potassium, phosphorus, magnesium, and iron. It has a high concentration of vitamins A, C, and K, and the phytonutrient sulforaphane—which studies at Johns Hopkins University suggest has powerful anti-cancer properties. Flax seeds are high in omega-3s. And avocados are full of good vitamins like B, A, and E, and good fat that makes for beautiful skin. Seeds and whole grains have protein, fiber, vitamin A, thiamin, riboflavin, niacin, vitamin B-12, folic acid, zinc, and iron. Tofu is rich in protein, fiber, vitamin A, thiamin, folic acid, calcium, zinc, iron, unsaturated fats, and anti-cancer phytonutrients. Tomatoes are no slouches either; they have vitamin A, vitamin C, carotenoids, especially lycopene. Not to mention all the good stuff in green leafy vegetables!

Kale, everyone's favorite superfood, is full of antioxidants, anti-inflammatory nutrients, and anti-cancer nutrients in the form of glucosinolates. The cancer preventative benefits in kale are from two types of antioxidants, carotenoids and flavonoids. And within the carotenoids, lutein and beta-carotene are the superstars. And, dig this: 100 calories of kale provide over 350 milligrams of the most basic omega-3 fatty acid (alpha-linolenic acid). Plants have plenty of protein and nutrients.

As for other animal proteins, like seafood, at least in the United States, always consult the *Monterey Bay Aquarium's Seafood Watch* to find out which fish is sustainably caught, and limit consumption of the big fish to three times a month. Currently, the oceans are poisoned with toxic chemicals and radiation. And the big fish, like tuna, swordfish, halibut, and even salmon, absorb all of that and more. Farmed fish are even worse, fed food colored with dyes, raised in polluted waters, prone to infection and disease. It's best to stick with eating things that have been on a mostly natural plant-based diet. I eat grass-fed beef five or six times a month, and occasionally I'll have shrimp or wild-caught Alaskan salmon, less now since the Fukushima nuclear disaster. Mostly, though, I enjoy legumes and plant proteins. They taste delicious, and they're really great for the body—lower in calories than animal proteins and with no saturated fat. Plus, my grocery bill is significantly lower.

But wait, you say, what about eggs? Aren't they high in protein? Yes, they are. Eggs are great. Eggs are easy to cook. Eggs make excellent dinners. Roasted tomato omelet, mushroom frittata, baked eggs with tomatoes and spinach, huevos rancheros, tacos with a fried egg, or poached eggs with a green salad. Dishes with eggs are among my favorite, an easy go-to dinner option. Here's the deal with eggs though, you must, for the good of your own health and the happiness of the egg laying chickens, buy only organic, pasture-raised. Talk to your grocer, check out the Farmers Market, or look at the list of purveyors on EatWild.com. Pasture-raised eggs are higher in vitamin E too. Eggs are a great source of protein. All B vitamins are found in eggs (vitamins B1, B2, B3, B5, B6, B12, choline, biotin, and folic acid). Choline is the big deal among these B vitamins. And, eggs rank higher in choline than most any other food. But, eggs have no fiber, and fiber is a necessity to any good diet. Eat your eggs with greens. You need fiber with that protein.

CHAPTER 19

FIBER KEEPS YOU AGELESS

Eat more fiber and you just may live longer.

A high fiber diet helps with weight loss. We all know that fiber is key to good health, but how do you know if you are getting enough? Most Americans aren't. The average adult only eats 15 grams of fiber per day. Everyone needs about 35-50 grams of fiber a day. It helps to normalize the body's blood sugar and insulin levels. Fiber lowers the risk of cardiovascular disease, diabetes, cancer, and other inflammatory-related diseases. Eat more plants. Best way to get more fiber.

Since we've been on the subjects of protein and fiber, let's talk tofu. Organic tofu is an almost perfect food. Those famous *Blue Zone* centenarians in Okinawa eat tofu daily. Their tofu is made locally, with no added chemicals or pesticides, and with organic soybeans. And they're over 100, healthy, strong, and content. Tofu is low in calories; it's high in protein and rich in minerals, and it even has some fiber. It has no cholesterol and it's eco-friendly, unlike beef or chicken. And here's even better news: tofu is complete in the amino acids necessary for human sustenance. Dan Buettner wrote a book called *The Blue Zones* about areas around the world where people live to be over 100, why they live this long, and how they maintain their health and happiness as they age. He praises tofu, which is a staple for the Japanese *Blue Zone* inhabitants, because it's "an excellent source of protein without the side effects of meat, tofu contains a compound, phytoestrogen, which may provide heart-protective properties to women." So, if you're concerned about tofu when it comes to estrogen mimicking effects, don't be. I've been asked by some of my Ageless Dieters about protein and the dangers of estrogen. Organic tofu is a safe and excellent alternative to meat. I love cooking with tofu. It's a key component in some of my most delicious meals. (Crispy baked tofu in a peanut sauce? Yes, please. And, the recipe is on our site!) Tofu is actually protective, not only in terms of heart-protective properties, but also for preventing cancer and the onset of early puberty.

In fact, there was a recent study and a book about the "new age of puberty" (girls developing earlier and earlier). Tofu was not the culprit for cancer or the onset of early puberty. In the study, it was found that the endocrine disrupting chemicals found in things like the plastics using Bisphenol A, or BPAs and in the antibiotics used in raising meat are triggering earlier development and puberty in girls. Antibiotics are used to make the animals get fatter and reach puberty faster, not just to protect against disease. Another good reason to buy organic, pasture-raised meats: no antibiotics. And BPA? It was actually invented as a medical estrogen, and it ended up in almost all plastics. BPA is also on paper, receipts, and in other compounds. Stay away from BPAs.

"The theory [about why tofu is good] would be that the estrogen mimicking effects of soy may actually cause the body to become resistant to estrogen—that it may down-regulate the estrogen receptor, so that later in life, your body doesn't perceive or see estrogen in quite the same way. We think that soy may actually be protective. The data is now coming out that women shouldn't worry so much about their soy intake for breast cancer, but it does speak to another concept in environmental health, which is the window of susceptibility. That means the timing of when you are exposed to something does affect the outcome. We think that children should eat soy because that's when it trains their body to become resistant to estrogen," says Louise Greenspan, co-author of *The New Puberty*, in an interview with Terry Gross on *Fresh Air*.

The other thing I love about tofu is that it adopts flavors beautifully. If you have a really flavorful marinade or sauce, it will take on those tastes. It's just really delectable in recipes. Bake it, grill it, or sauté it with a stir-fry. You can even use tofu in a vegan ceviche (raw because it's already "cooked" in the similar way of cheese).

Eating high-fiber foods keeps you feeling full. It's almost impossible to overeat if you eat enough fibrous foods at each meal. They fill you up and take longer to chew and give your brain time to get the signal you've eaten enough. Dietary fiber—found mainly in fruits, vegetables, whole grains and legumes—keeps you regular, relieves constipation, and is absolutely necessary for the health of your gut (and your microbiome). Foods containing fiber also provide other health benefits, helping to maintain a healthy weight, lowering your risk of diabetes and heart disease, controlling blood sugar levels, and contributing to a healthier, leaner body. For people with diabetes, fiber—particularly soluble fiber—slows the absorption of sugar and improves blood sugar levels. Scientists in microbiology and immunology and authors of *The Good Gut,* Justin and Erica Sonnenburg, urge us to eat plenty of fiber to nurture the delicate ecosystem of bacteria in your gut. The Standard American Diet, low in nutrition, high in processed foods, refined flours, conventional dairy, and sugar, is digested in the stomach and small intestine, and starves the microbes in your large intestine. And as the Sonnenburgs write, this has led to a "mass extinction event"—a calamity for our overall health, leading to what they suspect are more allergies, food and otherwise, and an alarming rise in obesity and autoimmune diseases. The beneficial bacteria have died off, making it much harder for our microbiota to play their role in cooling down inflammation, supporting our immune system, and helping us thrive. Their advice: stop sterilizing your home with antibacterial cleaning products and eat more fiber, which is digested by the bugs in your lower intestine.

What is fiber? The two types of fiber are soluble and insoluble. From the Mayo Clinic:

Soluble fiber. This type of fiber dissolves in water to form a gel-like material. It can help lower blood cholesterol and glucose levels. Soluble fiber is found in oats, peas, beans, apples, citrus fruits, carrots, barley and psyllium. [Legumes, fruits, nuts, seeds, omega-3 rich flaxseeds, chia seeds, and protein-rich hempseeds, cucumbers, celery, carrots, and in so many other plant-based foods and fruits have plenty of soluble fiber.]

Insoluble fiber. This type of fiber promotes the movement of material through your digestive system and increases stool bulk, so it can be of benefit to those who struggle with constipation or irregular stools. Nuts, beans and vegetables, such as cauliflower, green beans and potatoes, are good sources of insoluble fiber. [Millet, rye, barley, brown rice, lentils, chickpeas, kidney beans, carrots, Brussels sprouts, broccoli, kale and spinach are all great sources of insoluble fiber.]

Soluble fiber helps eliminate fat and lower cholesterol. Soluble fibers slow the rate at which sugars and fats enter your bloodstream. They've been shown to lower "bad" LDL cholesterol, especially for people with high cholesterol levels, when fed in large amounts.

All fiber—soluble and insoluble—is good fiber. Especially soluble fiber, which is necessary for weight loss and helps control cravings, because it fills you up and helps digestion. Bottom line: We need fiber to stay trim and ageless.

CHAPTER 20

EAT MORE OF THESE FOODS

"Life expectancy would grow by leaps and bounds if green vegetables smelled as good as bacon."
—DOUG LARSON

Fiber can help prevent obesity and all the chronic diseases related to aging. Here are a few more fiber facts: fiber is only present in plant foods. There is no fiber in any chicken, beef, fish, egg, or dairy products. Fiber is the part of plant foods your body can't digest. If you eat foods without fiber, like meat, eggs, and dairy, make sure to add fiber-rich foods to the meal. The more fiber a food has the better. Skip foods with added fiber; those products are processed, enriched and fortified. Stick with foods naturally high in fiber—fruits, vegetables, legumes, whole grains, nuts, and seeds. Fiber keeps you lean. Foods high in fiber tend to be naturally low-calorie, and fiber makes you feel fuller because it swells in the stomach when it absorbs liquid. Fibrous foods also tend to take longer to chew, giving the brain time to get the signal you're full. It has been shown in studies that people who consume 35-50 grams of fiber a day have more success with weight loss and lose the weight faster than those with lower fiber diets. They are simply less hungry from eating more fibrous foods. Fiber lowers blood pressure and glucose levels, and it increases blood flow. Fiber reduces inflammation in the body. Fiber keeps us regular and helps to prevent heart disease by reducing high blood pressure. People with high-fiber diets are much less likely to suffer from inflammatory illnesses, like diabetes and cancer, than someone on a low-fiber diet. Making high-fiber foods ageless foods.

How to get more fiber in your diet? Have a kale smoothie every day. Start by eating more fruits and vegetables, whole grains, nuts, flaxseeds, chia, hempseeds, and quinoa. Potatoes are a wonderful source of fiber. Other vegetables worth eating for fiber and phytonutrients are peas, artichokes, Brussels sprouts, broccoli, and kale. Berries, pears, and avocados are also high in fiber. Legumes are amazing sources of fiber. This includes split peas, lentils (super versatile, excellent in side dishes, as a main course, flavorful and delicious), black beans (among my favorite), and lima beans. All of these legumes have between 13-16 grams of fiber per cooked cup.

Eating more plant-based proteins that are high in fiber makes foods like quinoa damn near perfect. Quinoa is a complete protein, containing all nine essential amino acids, with twice as much fiber as other whole grains. Quinoa is a good source of folate. Like most other seeds, amaranth, chia, hemp, and buckwheat, quinoa is a good source of manganese, magnesium and phosphorus. One cup (185 grams) of quinoa has about 8 grams of protein and 5 grams of fiber per cup. If you eat quinoa regularly, this means you're getting a good dose of fiber and protein.

Hempseeds are an easily digestible plant protein, and 3 tablespoons gives you 11 grams of protein. They have a naturally perfect ratio of omega-3 fats, and those ageless minerals: magnesium, zinc, iron and phosphorus.

Chia seeds generate a lot of buzz these days, with good reason. They're high in many phytonutrients, fiber, and protein. Chia is an edible seed from the desert plant *Salvia hispanica*, dating back to the Aztec and Mayan heyday in Mexico. Chia seeds are full of healthy omega-3 fatty acids, carbohydrates, protein, fiber, antioxidants, and calcium. One ounce of chia seeds contains 4 grams of protein, 9 grams fat, 12 grams carbohydrates, 11 grams of fiber, and calcium, plus phytonutrients. Chia seeds are an easy food to add to smoothies, porridges, and sugar-free, vegan desserts. When soaked they form a gel and make for great pudding or jam.

Buckwheat is gluten-free grain high in protein and soluble fiber, which helps to slow down the rate of glucose absorption. It's good in porridges, salads, and savory dishes. Buckwheat protein is a balanced one, rich in lysine. Its amino acid score is 100—one of the highest amino acid scores among plant sources. It's rich in niacin, pantothenic acid, riboflavin, manganese, magnesium, phosphorus, copper, zinc and rutin, a powerful flavonoid. Rutin, an anti-inflammatory, as with other antioxidants, extends the power of vitamin C, and protects LDL cholesterol from oxidation.

To be ageless, follow the 4 Rules *and* eat more fiber.

CHAPTER 21

LIVE EXUBERANTLY, NOT MODERATELY

You are a perishable item, live accordingly.

The thing about a diet of moderation is that it will kill you. It will make you fat and sick and old. If you eat relatively well, it's not the 80 percent that makes you look and feel old, sick, and tired, it's that 20 percent. You can undo the good of a daily kale smoothie and a healthy lunch with a dinner of corn-fed steak, iceberg lettuce with blue cheese dressing, and a fat-free frozen yogurt. Everything in moderation is a whole lot of little bits of inflammatory foods that add up to a diet of toxins. This kind of diet is making Americans obese, sick, and biologically old. Stick with an anti-inflammatory diet and lifestyle, not a philosophy of "moderation in all things." Eat well, every day, all day, exercise regularly, meditate every day, and sleep immoderately, as much as you can.

I'll be straight with you: this diet is not one of moderation. A diet of moderation makes you sick, and a life of moderation would bore you. Moderation never created great works of art, amazing films, books, and buildings; moderation doesn't get you elected president or make you a CEO. Moderation doesn't even make you happy. Exuberance, enthusiasm, energized action, joy. These are not the words of a moderate person. Pursue what you love with gusto by eating and living for an ageless and vibrant you. **Eat clean and live out loud.**

What you eat informs your worldview and how you eat shapes your world. Do you eat the rainbow of fresh fruits and vegetables? Do you live in a colorful world? Or is your palate and, by extension, your life monochromatic and beige? Are you taking from the world or positively impacting the Earth? Eating more than 50 percent of food from animals takes a toll on this planet. If everyone lived the Paleo way, the decimation of land, water, plants and animals would be too big to bear. Eat lower on the food chain; eat more plants.

Are you energized? Imagine how your diet affects the spiritual side of your life. We hear a lot about the mind/body/spirit connection. They say yoga supports your mind, body, and spirit, as does meditation. But what does it mean? We understand the body and mind part of the trilogy, but what about the spirit? Our spirit is what moves us to live with joy. We get energy from food, and that energy powers our spirit. The power of food is great. It can heal our bodies, minds, and restore us to our core spiritual selves. Without a supple body and a strong mind we can lose sense of who we are spiritually. Yogi masters, philosophers from the East, have said this: *There is great power in food; 80 percent of the spiritual work is the food you eat. You want to make spiritual progress? You're almost there with a good diet.* Even if that's too much airy fairy talk for you, this fact is indisputable: food is the key. It's how we nourish our mind, body, and spirit.

So live immoderately, eat ageless.

CHAPTER 22

HYDRATE

Drinking water maintains the body's fluid balance.

Water is the source of life. Our bodies are 98 percent water. Drink water for maximum vibrancy. Part of being healthy is staying hydrated. *Hydrate.* Drink plenty of water all day, every day. You need more water than you think you do. Aim for *at least* 90 ounces a day, more if you exercise daily, and even more if it's a warm day and you're in the sun. I find I need at least 100 ounces a day. The Institute of Medicine recommends, in its general guidelines for water intake, that women consume a total of 91 ounces (that's about 2.7 liters) per day—from all food and beverages combined. And, for men, it's about 125 ounces a day (or 3.7 liters). I recommend more, if like me you're active throughout the day. I've discovered that a lot of the times I felt bad, suffered from a stomach ache, cramps, fatigue, headaches or migraines, distended belly or constipation, I was dehydrated. Nowadays, if I have a headache, I drink two big glasses of water first and then wait and see. Usually I feel much better. By the time you feel thirsty, you're already dehydrated. Don't wait for thirst to signal the need to drink water, get ahead of the game and hydrate all day. Buy yourself a really good, BPA-free water bottle and take it everywhere you go. I have one I travel with, and fill up before each flight. Airports, some yoga studios, and gyms now have those really convenient filtered water fountains designed specifically for water bottles.

Daily symptoms like fatigue, lethargy, headaches, inability to focus, dizziness, nausea, stomach aches or cramps, and lack of strength are all possible signs of dehydration. If you feel tired, nauseous, headache-y, drink a big glass of water. In fact when in doubt, drink a glass or bottle of water. Proper hydration is a necessity for good digestion, a healthy body and brain, and great looking skin. If you want to look ageless and have luminous skin, drink plenty of filtered water. Always, always turn to water before you reach for juice (more sugar in a glass of juice than a candy bar which requires MORE water to digest!), a so-called health drink (also, often full of sugars or sugar substitutes), or soft drinks. Soft drinks, flavored waters, caffeinated drinks, and alcohol will dehydrate you.

My advice: start every day with a big glass of water. Before coffee, before the berry smoothie, I drink two 12-ounce glasses of water. I feel better than the old days of coffee first, water much later. You will start your day in a much better way if you begin with water. Squeeze a little fresh lemon juice for added sweetness and flavor. Hydrating when you wake, 20 minutes before drinking or consuming anything else, is a good thing to do because water with lemon oxygenates and energizes the body. This jumpstarts your metabolism by stimulating the stomach to increase its production of digestive juices. It improves peristalsis (the muscular contractions that push food through the entire digestive system), which means improved digestion, which in turn leads to better nutrient absorption. This means less bloating. Drinking a glass of water with lemon first thing stimulates the liver's production of bile. This helps with waste removal, keeps you regular, and it also acts as a mild diuretic, helping to gently flush out toxins from the urinary tract. So tomorrow, try a new wake-up routine: start with a very big glass of filtered water with fresh lemon (or lime) juice.

Avoid plain old tap water unless you're living in a pristine mountain town, and invest in a good filtration system. Most tap water has aluminum and arsenic in it. Neither of those is good for you. In fact, aluminum has been shown to contribute to Alzheimer's. And arsenic, well, we know arsenic is a poison. The level of arsenic in most U.S. tap water is high. Arsenic is a powerful carcinogenic, which has been linked to an increased risk of the development of several types of cancer. The Natural Resources Defense Council estimates as many as 56 million Americans living in 25 states drink water with arsenic at unsafe levels. As we degrade our environment, expect drinking water to become less and less drinkable and more and more poisonous. Most community waters are treated with Disinfection Byproducts (DBPs) and chlorine to clean the water. And skip the bottled water, most bottled water is either obtained at great expense to the natural world or it's plain old tap water. Some estimate that 40 percent of popular bottled waters sold are filled with tap water. Yep, that's right. So get yourself a good BPA free water bottle, save yourself serious money, and refill that bottle regularly with filtered or spring water. The best option money and health wise is filtered tap water. It's also the most environmentally sound choice you can make. Install a water filter for your home, your office, and try to stick to filtered water wherever you go. It's easier and easier these days. Most gyms, restaurants, airports, and public spaces have filtered water fountains.

Bottom line: stay hydrated; drink filtered tap water.

CHAPTER 23

COOL DOWN INFLAMMATION. JUST SAY NO TO IN-FLAMMATORY DISEASES & ALZHEIMER'S

What you eat can either fuel or cool down inflammation.

A big reason I started living ageless is that by staying free of inflammation, which causes lifestyle diseases and triggers infections, I could prevent Alzheimer's. This was a serious concern because my grandmother, one of my all-time favorite people, died of Alzheimer's. It was brutal and ruthless. Alzheimer's destroyed her mind, her body, and broke my grandfather's heart. For me feeling good and losing weight and inflammation are great, but it's the side effect of preventing inflammatory, lifestyle-related diseases like Alzheimer's that keeps me really happy.

This is supported by serious science. It is absolutely possible to prevent Alzheimer's and other diseases by changing your diet and lifestyle, by cooling down inflammation. Teams of scientists and researchers have discovered the diseases and ailments most people suffer from as they age ultimately affect the brain, sending the immune cells into high alert. High alert is a hyperactive, destructive state. These ailments are caused by an inflammatory lifestyle and diet (little exercise, sleep deprivation, and a diet rich in processed foods, excessive animal proteins, wheat, dairy, and sugar). "'The idea is simple: monitoring and prompt treatment [of inflammation] could prevent the decline from Alzheimer's,' said Hugh Perry of the University of Southampton, UK, as he presented the research at the Alzheimer's Research UK annual meeting in Oxford," from an article in *New Science* by Andy Coghlan.

Even if you don't care about Alzheimer's or worry about getting one of these lifestyle diseases, this diet is one of the best options for preventing premature aging. If avoiding disease isn't your primary concern, that's fine, I understand. Consider this: how your skin, hair, and nails look give you an idea of what is happening internally. The external is a serious signpost for internal health. If you have prematurely aged skin, brittle hair and nails you are probably deficient in key nutrients. You want your skin to glow, give it what it needs to produce collagen and healthy connective tissue. Cool down inflammation, feel and see the difference in your body.

CHAPTER 24

FOODS TO EAT
FOR MAXIMUM
AGELESSNESS

"People who love to eat are always the best people."
—JULIA CHILD

I've written a lot about the foods that spell early death, disease, and destruction—foods that lead to premature aging. We know what they are now: processed foods and drinks, sugar, wheat, and dairy. Following Ageless Rule #1 we drop these ticking time bombs from our diet. And now, it's time to focus on the true key to success. Focus on ALL the amazing foods we CAN and WILL be eating (a full shopping list is in the back of this book, with cooking tips, meal plans, and recipes). These are foods that heal, foods that taste good and energize you.

Anti-inflammatory, often low-glycemic, fruits and vegetables are a great start towards eating for agelessness. This includes plants like kale, broccoli, spinach, carrots, cantaloupe, cherries, and sweet potatoes. They contain carotenoids that protect against DNA damage—keeping those wonderful telomeres nice and long! But, this isn't a raw foods diet. You'll be doing magical things to these plants, enhancing their natural goodness and flavor. And there are plenty of good fats to make food taste even better and help to protect DNA from oxidative damage. Plant-based fats including extra-virgin olive oil, coconut oil, avocado oil, hemp oil, walnut oil, sesame oil, and flaxseed oil are serious flavor enhancers. We are lucky there are so many foods out there that are naturally flavorful and good for us. There are phytochemicals in black, green, and white teas that inhibit DNA damage. And, herbs! Fresh herbs enhance any dish, and they contain incredibly powerful antioxidants and anti-aging, anti-inflammatory compounds. Among my favorite go-to herbs are basil, parsley, mint, cilantro, oregano, thyme, rosemary, and tarragon. I could make a big salad of just herbs. In fact, during the summer, I often do. They add big flavor to anything you're making from smoothies to omelets to Thai basil beef.

Garlic! I'm a huge fan. Garlic imparts great flavor to dishes, and it's a major antioxidant. Garlic is mouth-wateringly good in vinaigrettes, Caesar salads, soups, hummus, carne asada, black beans, roasted chicken, and so many other wonderful recipes. Besides tasting good raw, sautéed, baked, or grilled, garlic neutralizes free radicals present in blood. It helps the heart muscle stay strong and healthy. Obviously, you want a strong heart, powering you to create the life you desire.

And tasty fruits like berries of all colors, with their flavonoids, have serious antioxidant and anti-inflammatory effects. They're wonderful by themselves or in other dishes like chia pudding, berry desserts, as part of a big fruit salad, or on their own. A dish of ripe berries can be the ultimate treat on a hot summer day. Begin your morning with a berry smoothie, or as my friend Todd calls it, "berries in a glass," and your day will start right.

The more you eat of these good plants, the better you'll feel, the sharper your mind will be, and the better you'll look.

And nuts! Filled with good fiber and protein, fat-packed nuts are great. Try to eat only organic, whole, and unprocessed nuts. They may cost a little more, but there is a reason you don't want to buy Class B eggs from a grocer. Buy higher quality ingredients, you're paying it forward. Nuts like cashews and peanuts are often contaminated with mold. My favorite nuts are almonds, macadamias, Brazil nuts, pine nuts, and walnuts. I eat nuts in the morning with my detox smoothie if I'm too rushed to have a proper sit-down breakfast. And, I'm energized and satiated for hours. Nuts affect several genes that control tumor growth, metabolism, cutting cancer risk and slowing growth of tumors. And they have been known to contribute to better brain function. When your energy dips at around 2:00 p.m. drink your kale smoothie and eat a few nuts.

Both the body (your gut!) and brain love fiber, which means we do too! If you want to be ageless remember those 35-50 grams of fiber the body needs every day. Drink your kale smoothie, eat your veggies, and cook yourself black beans and rice for supper. For me, this 10-minute meal always hits the spot. And who doesn't have 10-15 minutes to cook themselves dinner?

Fiber helps to normalize the body's insulin levels. And your insulin levels are the dominant factor in obesity. David S. Ludwig, director of the New Balance Foundation Obesity Prevention Center at Boston Children's Hospital and a professor of pediatrics at Harvard Medical School, and Mark I. Friedman, vice president of research at the Nutrition Science Initiative, wrote about this in *The New York Times* opinion section. They explained why some people are always hungry, even when they're overweight and overeating. "Many biological factors affect the storage of calories in fat cells, including genetics, levels of physical activity, sleep and stress. But one has an indisputably dominant role: the hormone insulin. We know that excess insulin treatment for diabetes causes weight gain, and insulin deficiency causes weight loss. And of everything we eat, highly refined and rapidly digestible carbohydrates produce the most insulin. High consumption of refined carbohydrates— chips, crackers, cakes, soft drinks, sugary breakfast cereals and even white rice and bread—has increased body weights throughout the population." Fiber, from fruits, vegetables, whole grains, legumes, nuts and seeds, is integral in normalizing insulin levels and in reducing body weight. The fresh foods that are high in fiber are also often high in nutrition. Great sources of fiber include legumes (if you love chickpeas, good news, they're very high in fiber). I love legumes because they're flavorful, versatile, nutrient-packed, and easy to cook. They really are the best. Black beans, adzuki beans, kidney beans, chickpeas, navy beans, lentils, cannellini or white beans, edamame, great northern beans, lima beans, pinto beans, soybeans, white beans, black-eyed peas, cowpeas, pigeon peas, split peas, soy and fermented soy products—soybeans, miso, tempeh, tofu, and mung bean sprouts. I could eat mung bean sprouts in everything, especially with spaghetti squash in place of rice noodles with a lime peanut sauce. Discover your favorite legumes and incorporate them into your diet. There are so many great recipes using beans, chickpeas, soy, and sprouts. I sometimes think I'm obsessed with legumes. And, it's a healthy obsession. It's clean food and it's affordable.

Fiber is necessary for a healthy gut and for happy gut bacteria. And a healthy gut is vital. If you have a healthy gut, you're healthier, mentally and physically, and you're leaner. Gut bacteria produce molecules (called short chain fatty acids) that promote the growth of other beneficial bacteria and archaea. What's archaea? "Although most research has focused on gut bacteria, current evidence suggests that the Archaea—an ancient domain of single-celled organisms—are resident within the gut in high numbers, and have direct and indirect effects on the host." From a study published in Nature.com. You want happy beneficial bacteria and archaea, eat your fiber-rich fruits and vegetables. And, "the more fiber you feed these friendly inhabitants, the more types of species appear, studies have found. This bump in microbial diversity has been linked to a slimmer waistline. 'Undigested carbohydrates allow the whole ecosystem to thrive and flourish,' Purna Kashyap, a gastroenterologist at the Mayo Clinic in Rochester, Minn. says." From an article for NPR's *The Salt* blog by Michaeleen Doucleff.

Whole grains and pseudocereals are adaptable in dishes and can be quite delicious, and they are loaded with plenty of good fiber and protein. These include: brown rice, amaranth, millet, steel-cut oats, quinoa (though, technically a seed), buckwheat (which is, despite its misleading name, gluten-free). Fiber rich starches that are full of phytonutrients, including sweet potatoes, the squashes (butternut, kabocha, spaghetti, acorn), fresh corn, green peas, can be delicious on their own or as part of a hearty meal, and they keep you feeling satiated. These kinds of starches are ideal for when you need energy! Starches have valuable calcium, iron, B vitamins and fiber.

There was an illuminating article in *The New York Times* by Jo

Robinson (of EatWild.com) about how we've bred the nutrients out of conventional vegetables, and how to find plants that are still nutrient rich. We've been doing this for centuries because humans wanted sweeter, less bitter fruits and vegetables. But the good news is that there are still plenty of foods available at the Farmers Market and grocery stores with abundant nutrients and flavor. We just need to be more cognizant of which fruits and vegetables have more good stuff in them. Ms. Robinson writes, "If we want to get maximum health benefits from fruits and vegetables, we must choose the right varieties. Studies published within the past 15 years show that much of our produce is relatively low in phytonutrients, which are the compounds with the potential to reduce the risk of four of our modern scourges: cancer, cardiovascular disease, diabetes and dementia. The loss of these beneficial nutrients did not begin 50 or 100 years ago, as many assume. Unwittingly, we have been stripping phytonutrients from our diet since we stopped foraging for wild plants some 10,000 years ago and became farmers."

Eat more weeds! Eat more Arugula, watercress, scallions (the green and white parts), fresh herbs, including cilantro, basil, parsley, and mint, and add more garlic to your food. These plants have not had the phytonutrients bred out of them. Choose plants with dark colors, greens, reds, oranges, and purples. Skip the iceberg lettuce and sweet corn (unless it's July and your Farmers Market has a bumper crop—there are few things finer than summer corn, fresh-from-the-garden tomatoes, and basil), and join my arugula and watercress fan club. Those spicy, peppery greens are intensely flavorful. Take Ms. Robinson's advice and try dandelion greens. They're sold almost everywhere, or you could harvest them from your backyard (provided your soil is organic). And if you find that dandelion greens are too bitter for you in the raw, try them in an omelet with scallions and roasted tomatoes, or in salad with a little sweetness from basil, fresh corn, roasted carrots, cherry tomatoes, and a lovely vinaigrette. I add dandelion greens to my detox smoothies. I don't even taste the bitterness thanks to the other good stuff in the smoothie. Writes Ms. Robinson, "Wild dandelions, once a springtime treat for Native Americans, have seven times more phytonutrients than spinach, which we consider a 'superfood.' A purple potato native to Peru has 28 times more cancer-fighting anthocyanins than common russet potatoes." Choose arugula over lettuce. Arugula, or rocket, is rich in the cancer-fighting compounds glucosinolates. And it's higher in antioxidant activity, which promotes agelessness.

She writes that, "Scallions, or green onions, are jewels of nutrition hiding in plain sight. They resemble wild onions and are just as good for you. Remarkably, they have more than five times more phytonutrients than many common onions do. The green portions of scallions are more nutritious than the white bulbs, so use the entire plant. Herbs are wild plants incognito. We've long valued them for their intense flavors and aroma, which is why they've not been given a flavor makeover. Because we've left them well enough alone, their phytonutrient content has remained intact." Load up on basil, parsley, mint, and cilantro. I love fresh herbs and use them in everything from my kale smoothie to burgers. Once you know what to eat, (fresh vegetables, greens, grass-fed beef, fresh pasture-raised eggs, organic tofu, nuts, berries, prepared with olive, sesame, and coconut oils), it's easy to create an Ageless Diet that suits your palate.

As you add more fresh vegetables, legumes, and grains, start to decrease your meat consumption. Ideally, you're moving towards an 80 percent plant-based diet. Better for you, better for the Earth. And plants can be so flavorful. Alain Passard, world-renowned French chef, has, since 2001, taken meat off the menu at his very famous restaurant to focus his passion on vegetables. And, chefs from around the world have taken notice, flocking to his restaurant L'Arpége. Why? Because Chef Passard's food tastes delicious, it's exciting because vegetables can have an almost infinite flavor profile. "'There is a creativity with vegetables that you don't have with animal tissue," he explains. *La cuisine végétale* offers the chef "a tremendous amount of surprises, because there is still everything to be done with a tomato, a carrot, an eggplant. There is a lot of enchantment in vegetable cookery. And," he adds, "it is totally transparent.'" From an interview with the great chef in *Bon Appétit* by Christine Muhlke. Given his genius for creating edible masterpieces with plants, it's no surprise that the chef is ruled by the seasons.

And, he says it makes the dishes even more memorable, more magical. "When you really respect the seasons, it works all by itself."

According to Dr. Campbell in his book *The China Study,* "People who ate the most animal-based foods got the most chronic disease. People who ate the most plant-based foods were the healthiest. Caldwell B. Esselstyn, Jr., M.D., a physician and researcher at the best cardiac center in the country, The Cleveland Clinic, treated 18 patients with established coronary disease with a 100 percent whole food, mostly plant-based diet. Not only did the intervention stop the progression of the disease but 70 percent of the patients also saw an opening of their clogged arteries. Dr. Dean Ornish, a graduate of Harvard Medical School, completed a similar study with consistent results."

Dr. Campbell writes that, "There are virtually no nutrients in animal-based foods that are not better provided by plants." Protein, fiber, vitamins, minerals—you name it, they've got it, and the health benefits.

What you put in your mouth shapes your values and beliefs about the world you inhabit. Are you living in a colorful, rich, magical world? Is this one that supports and nourishes you?

CHAPTER 25

EAT FOR A HAPPY GUT

"All disease begins in the gut."
—HIPPOCRATES

"When in doubt treat the gut."
—MARK CARNEY, ND, LAc

Are you eating foods that encourage easeful digestion? If not, start today. It's key for good health. You digest the world through your gut. There's serious truth to the idea that the gut is your sixth sense. "The gut can work independently of any control by the brain in your head—it's functioning as a second brain," says Michael Gershon, professor and chair of pathology and cell biology at Columbia. "It's another independent center of integrative neural activity." Seek out an anti-inflammatory diet that sustains a healthy gut and encourages optimal health.

When you eat for a healthy gut you have much more energy. Scientists say we are as much *we*—our bodies, organs, blood, and DNA—as we are bacteria. "There are 10 times more bacterial cells in your body than human cells, according to Carolyn Bohach, a microbiologist at the University of Idaho," from Melinda Wenner of *Scientific American*.

If you are eating mostly processed foods, pesticide-sprayed produce, hormone and antibiotic pumped meats, genetically modified foods, what are you telling your gut about the world? Your gut, *your microbiome*, responds to the information you give it, and this means the food you feed it and the environment you live in. To paraphrase Steve Jobs, a strong gut (intuition) is more powerful than intelligence. Emotion and intuition are rooted in the "second brain"—the gut.

Take care of the beneficial bacteria, and they will take care of you. Intestinal bacteria produce chemicals that help you harness energy and nutrients from food; they keep the immune system healthy. And they are a vital in looking and feeling ageless.

The human body is made up of trillions of cells, and the microbiome harbors a hundred trillion bacteria. For every gene in the genome, there are one hundred bacterial ones. This is the **microbiome**, and the impact it has on the body's health and ability to digest and absorb food is massive. Be conscious of what you feed these friendly critters.

Michael Pollan, author of *In Defense of Food*, wrote about the microbiome in *The New York Times Magazine*: "Justin Sonnenburg, a microbiologist at Stanford, suggests that we would do well to begin regarding the human body as 'an elaborate vessel optimized for the growth and spread of our microbial inhabitants.' This humbling new way of thinking about the self has large implications for human and microbial health, which turn out to be inextricably linked. Disorders in our internal ecosystem—a loss of diversity, say, or a proliferation of the 'wrong' kind of microbes—may predispose us to obesity and a whole range of chronic diseases, as well as some infections. Our resident microbes also appear to play a critical role in training and modulating our immune system, helping it to accurately distinguish between friend and foe and not go nuts on, well, nuts and all sorts of other potential allergens. Some researchers believe that the alarming increase in autoimmune diseases in the West may owe to a disruption in the ancient relationship between our bodies and their 'old friends'—the microbial symbionts with whom we coevolved."

Now, I'm not anti-antibiotics or anti-vaccines, but I'd prefer they stayed out of my food. Obviously, we never want to go back to the time before antibiotics. They are lifesaving, and we are lucky to have access. But do we need to take a preventative course of antibiotics every time we get a cold? Do we need all soap to be "anti-bacterial?" And, do we really need so many pesticides in our foods? Pesticides destroy good gut microbes and foster bad ones. Another

good reason to eat mostly organic foods, if you don't care about all
the bees dying, care about your own bugs.

And, you certainly want a finely tuned "gut instinct," right?
Well, again, it goes back to the friendly bacteria in your gut.

Mr. Pollan, in his research, discovered this: "Our gut bacteria
also play a role in the manufacture of substances like neurotrans-
mitters (including serotonin); enzymes and vitamins (notably Bs
and K) and other essential nutrients (including important amino
acid and short-chain fatty acids); and a suite of other signaling molecules that talk to, and influence, the immune and the metabolic
systems. Some of these compounds may play a role in regulating
our stress levels and even temperament: when gut microbes from
easygoing, adventurous mice are transplanted into the guts of anxious and timid mice, they become more adventurous. The expression 'thinking with your gut' may contain a larger kernel of truth
than we thought."

All right, a healthy gut is of paramount importance, so how do
we keep the beneficial bacteria happy?

One way to foster a healthier gut is to eat more naturally fermented foods. As Sandor Katz, author of *The Art of Fermentation,*
puts it, "Fermentation is the transformative action of micro-organisms. . . . not every transformative action results in something delicious that we want to put in our mouths," but often, it does. Pickles,
sauerkraut, miso, beer, wine . . . all delicious results of fermentation. And, guess what? Your gut loves fermented foods. Lately I've
been eating more of them, and I can feel a difference. My digestion
is better, and my immune system is stronger. I really enjoy the tastes
of fermented foods; they're tangy and flavorful. Fermentation adds
depth and complexity to foods. I love using Nama Shoyu soy sauce
and miso paste to flavor soups, dressings, sauces and marinades for
meats, fermented vegetables, long-ferment breads, and, of course,
biodynamic wine and dark organic beer.

If you're not gluten intolerant, and you're past the first 28 days
on the *Reset,* find a bakery making bread that's naturally (slow-
rise) fermented. I'm a particular fan of the whole wheat sourdough
bread from a bakery in Carbondale, Colorado. I sometimes buy it

in the summer at the Aspen Farmers Market. This bakery, and others around the country embracing artisanal, slow-food movement bread baking, ferment their dough with wild yeasts for at least 12-15 hours, often for at least 24 hours. This improves the digestibility of the bread and lowers its glycemic index, helping to keep blood sugar levels low. The bakery in Carbondale uses "whole-milled" whole wheat flour, meaning flour that's been milled from its intact state. And, the long-fermented sourdough I love has the bacteria *Lactobacillus* in a higher proportion to yeast than do other breads. More *Lactobacillus* means higher production of lactic acid, which means less phytic acid. This gives you the more mineral availability and easier digestion, made possible by the bacteria-yeast combo working to predigest the starches in the grains.

Naturally fermented pickled vegetables (which have naturally occurring probiotics), include kosher dill pickles, sauerkraut, pickled onions, carrots, and beets are also great. Maybe because I'm from South Carolina I have a thing for pickled foods. They're irresistible, and my gut is grateful.

Naturally fermented foods are relatively easy to find. You want organic fermented foods made with no preservatives. Real, fermented pickles and sauerkraut are worlds apart from most of the pickles you find in the condiment aisle of the average store. Real pickles are kept in your grocer's refrigerated section, and their list of ingredients is very simple: cucumbers or cabbage, water, salt, garlic and spices. And they don't contain vinegar. Why not? Because naturally fermented "real" pickles and sauerkraut create their own acids as they ferment. These are the probiota, the beneficial microbes that provide additional nutrients, aid digestion, and are beloved by your microbiome. They offer a wide range of additional health benefits, including reducing the risk for cancer. Nowadays most natural food stores and Farmers Markets sell naturally fermented foods—artisanal pickles abound at the New York City Union Square Farmers Market. Or, you can buy them online. (We have a list of our favorites on AgelessDietLife.com.) For a late lunch or snack, I'll have a piece of toasted long-fermented sourdough bread with half an avocado, sea salt, and one sliced *Bubbies* garlicky kosher dill pickle on top. It tastes so good, and if I really want to gild the lily, I'll put a mound of alfalfa sprouts on top of that.

As Mr. Pollan learned, what you feed your gut matters. "And the key to feeding the fermentation in the large intestine is giving it lots of plants with their various types of fiber, including resistant starch (found in bananas, oats, beans); soluble fiber (in onions and other root vegetables, nuts); and insoluble fiber (in whole grains, especially bran, and avocados). With our diet of swiftly absorbed sugars and fats we're eating for one and depriving the trillion of the food they like best: complex carbohydrates and fermentable plant fibers. The byproduct of fermentation is the short-chain fatty acids that nourish the gut barrier and help prevent inflammation. And there are studies suggesting that just by simply adding plants to a fast-food diet it can mitigate its inflammatory effect."

Eating ageless is the easiest way to keep your microbiome flourishing.

Good gut health is one of the reasons I try to buy only organic. If you can, I highly recommend it. And if you're worried about the extra money being spent, think about how we rarely hesitate to spend money on dinners out, lunches on the go, processed foods, or other "treats." Look at how much we're willing to spend on car or house maintenance. Body maintenance has got to be as important as your car's health, right? Maintaining the good health of our bodies is probably the most important thing you can do. If you don't have good health, a strong, vital microbiome, what do you have? So, buy as many fresh foods that are free of pesticides as possible.

Journalist and writer Lisa Garber investigated the damage pesticides and herbicides, like Roundup, do to our overall health in her article for *Natural Society*: many of us "forget the gut when it comes to warding off the flu and other more threatening diseases, but the gut—and its army of beneficial bacteria—are essential in protecting us from harm. That's why eating genetically modified and/or conventionally farmed food could be a direct assault on your own health. Most recently, research has shown that Monsanto's herbicide, known as Roundup, is destroying gut health, threatening overall health of animals, people, and the planet significantly. The journal *Current Microbiology* recently published a study that caught Monsanto's Roundup herbicide active ingredient, glyphosate, suppressing beneficial bacteria in poultry specimens. Given that gut health is directly linked to chronic illnesses and overall health" we would be smart to limit our exposure to pesticides, insecticides, herbicides, and genetically modified foods.

What can you do to avoid all of these nasty things added to food? Drop the Dirty Dozen™ when buying produce. The Environmental Working Group (EWG) keeps an updated list on the Dirty Dozen. This organization of scientists, researchers and policymakers created a list, guiding consumers on which foods are best bought organic—those on the Dirty Dozen list. Sticking with organic on the Dirty Dozen reduces the amount of toxins you consume on a daily basis by as much as 80 percent. They put together two lists, *The Dirty Dozen* and *The Clean 15,* one for when to buy organic, and the other, when you can safely purchase the cheaper, conventionally grown produce.

The Dirty Dozen **Plus** List in 2015:

1. Apples

2. Peaches

3. Nectarines

4. Strawberries

5. Grapes

6. Celery

7. Spinach

8. Sweet bell peppers

9. Cucumbers

10. Cherry tomatoes

11. Snap peas (imported)

12. Potatoes

Plus these vegetables, which may contain organophosphate insecticides, and the EWG characterizes these as "highly toxic" and of special concern:

1. Kale/collard greens

2. Hot peppers (jalapeños, Serrano, etc.)

And the Clean 15 (foods with the least amount of pesticides):

1. Avocados

2. Sweet corn

3. Pineapples

4. Cabbage

5. Sweet peas (frozen)

6. Onions

7. Asparagus

8. Mangos

9. Papayas

10. Kiwi

11. Eggplant

12. Grapefruit

13. Cantaloupe

14. Cauliflower

15. Sweet potatoes

Dr. Andrew Weil says this about the EWG and pesticides: "The EWG points out that there is a growing consensus in the scientific community that small doses of pesticides and other chemicals can have adverse effects on health, especially during vulnerable periods such as fetal development and childhood." Pesticides also eradicate beneficial bacteria in your gut. If they're designed to kill bugs that eat growing plants, I would imagine they could be just as efficient in killing our own bugs, the bugs that help us digest plants for our nutrition.

Bottom line: take care of your gut and your gut will definitely take care of you. Eat a diverse, colorful diet, full of organic fruits, vegetables, legumes, seeds, whole grains, plenty of fiber, and seek out naturally fermented foods.

CHAPTER 26

CLEANSE & RESET

**You are what you eat.
So don't be fast, easy, cheap, or fake.**

*"If we could give every individual the right amount
of nourishment and exercise, not too little and not too much,
we would have found the safest way to health."*

—HIPPOCRATES

The *Reset* is 6 weeks, and the first week of that reset is the *Cleanse*. It's an easy way to reboot the system, get rid of impurities in your body, and lose the initial inflammation quickly. This cleanse is not one of those extreme Madonna or Beyoncé cleanses, and it's not the Master Cleanse. But you will get clean—clean of toxins and addictive substances. You won't go hungry and you will enjoy flavorful, satisfying foods. For these first 7 days, you'll have two tasty detox smoothies, a healthy lunch with greens and legumes or tofu, plant-based proteins, and then a healthy dinner with lean protein, great salads, delicious sauces, and plenty of water. You stop eating by 6:00 p.m. every day, for the first week. That's right, your last meal of the day is before 6:00 p.m.. *No food after 6:00.* This gives your body time to digest your evening meal. It also takes away any temptation, especially for those of us who sometimes snack while watching TV. It's also harder to burn those calories consumed later in the day, as you get closer to bedtime. You'll sleep better too. So, for this first week, stop all eating by 6:00 p.m.. If you work late, make sure you have a big hearty, ageless lunch.

For the full 7 days, give up coffee, alcohol, sugar, dairy, wheat, and some whole grains. If you're worried about caffeine withdrawal, don't be, you can have green tea (matcha is the most power-packed). And you'll be feeling so energized from the morning detox smoothie, the supplements, and your new, improved lifestyle, you won't miss the coffee. It's a terrific way to kickstart your *Reset* and the next 5 weeks.

Several years ago, I would buy 4 boules a week, a dense sourdough bread with a crispy crust in the shape of a small ball, from Whole Foods. Every night Scott and I would share half a loaf of this bread with a bowl of olive oil on the side for dipping. Afterwards, we'd enjoy a cookie or two—organic, home-baked. Scott regularly had asthma attacks, rather severe ones, and I was mainlining Benadryl. We were inflamed. And it didn't really matter how much we worked out, we always had a little extra flab around the belly. No matter how many crunches I did daily, and I did hundreds, I still had that little potbelly. No matter how many reps with 5-pound weights I did in yoga sculpt daily I never got toned arms. I couldn't understand it. Our wheat and sugar consumption was in relative moderation, a kale smoothie in the afternoon, a post-dinner cookie here and there, half a loaf of fresh-baked bread with a nice chunk of cheese, and a sensible dinner at night. A diet well within most people's concept of healthy, but we were still bigger than we wanted *and* not as healthy as we could have been. We certainly didn't really look or feel 100 percent ageless. We were eating sugar, wheat, and dairy in moderation. We had the perfect everything-in-moderation-diet. And it showed; we were moderately flabby with somewhat splotchy skin. We had no idea what the issue was for us . . . was it the dairy, the added sugar, the bread, the late dinners out at restaurants, the beer and wine? We needed a cleanse and reset to discover what worked and didn't work for our bodies. And we needed more than a few weeks to make those changes stick, and to develop new habits that would keep us healthy and lean.

Subtract all the inflammatory foods so you can discover what the biggest allergens are for you. We're all different. For me, dairy upsets my digestion and triggers sinus headaches. For Scott, it's wheat, but not steel-cut oats or sprouted whole grains containing gluten. We're all different, yet we share allergens to a lot of the same foods. Foods that are mass-produced, processed, stripped of nutrients end up being highly inflammatory substances—foods for an AGED diet.

Why do the *Reset* for 6 weeks? For a clean slate. In order to accurately understand what triggers inflammation for you, it is essential to bring the body back to a baseline by eating clean for a period that is long enough to allow your body to eliminate any current irritants. Without the initial *7-Day Cleanse* you may continue to live in a low grade inflammatory state for the rest of your life. And without the full *6 Week Reset*, you won't have the time and space to adopt better habits and to learn how to incorporate the Ageless Diet in your life. So what is it for you? Is it dairy? Are you one of 50 million and counting who have intolerance to lactose giving you digestive issues, bad skin, and congestion? Is it gluten? Can you easily digest steel-cut oats, bulgur wheat, spelt, farro, freekeh, and other grains with gluten? Can you drink beer? Or do grains containing gluten inflame you? You will know what works for you and what doesn't after the first 28 days.

And after those first 4 weeks, you'll have 2 more weeks to fit this new way of living into your daily life. It takes a full 6 weeks to really make these changes stick. Make sure you give yourself that time and space. It's the best thing I ever did for myself. I like me better. I'm brighter, happier, healthier, and I think you will be too. *Cleanse, Reset . . . Ageless.*

CHAPTER 27

AGELESS RULES

*"If we're not willing to settle for junk living,
we certainly shouldn't settle for junk food."*
—SALLY EDWARDS

It's really simple. **4 Ageless Rules**. Eat right, sleep, exercise, and meditate. Nothing about this is too time consuming or expensive. Everything you need to know for maximum agelessness is here in this book. This is your toolkit. You can easily live this way for the rest of your life, tweaking the Rules to fit your busy lifestyle. But, it does require a commitment. Do you want to fix your diet, change your life and feel great, or do you want to keep doing what you're doing, aging into a fatter, sicker body? It's up to you. What else have you got to do with your life than take care of you? Sure, work, build a career, raise the kids, support the family, hang out with friends, and travel. But without a healthy, whole YOU, work and everything else won't happen. Meet the challenges of your life feeling the best you can.

"Change your diet, change your life."
—TANIA VAN PELT

And, it all starts with the *6 Week Reset*. Those first 7 days on the *Cleanse* are critical. It prepares you for the rest of the 6 weeks.

I promise you'll have plenty to eat for the whole 6 weeks, and especially for those first 7 days of the *Cleanse*, and you'll have the added support of extra nutrients—essential vitamins and minerals, antioxidants. You'll have supplements to support your new diet and lifestyle and supplements for extra energy, better health, and deeper sleep. Commit to the *Cleanse* and *Reset*. Commit to feeling better and looking ageless.

After the first 7 days (a menu and meal plans for the *Cleanse* are in the back of this book), you can add a few more whole, intact grains, alcohol (stick with organic/biodynamic wines) in moderation, and coffee (organic only, preferably free-trade). You can also eat after 6:00 p.m., though if it feels good to have your last meal of the day by 6:00 p.m., then stick with this rule. Do what works for you and your biorhythm.

For the full 6 weeks no added sugars, sugar substitutes, no processed foods.

For the first 3 weeks drop ALL dairy from your diet.

After the first 3 weeks, you can introduce a little grass-fed, pasture-raised organic dairy (stick with goat milk cheese—easier for the body to digest). Observe how your body reacts to this allergen. Are you feeling congested? How are you digesting it? If there are any issues, quit eating it. And, because dairy is a known inflammatory food for almost everyone, it's best if you seriously limit your consumption.

For the first 28 days stop eating wheat, and all grains and foods that have gluten in them (www.celiac.com is a great resource to find out which foods contain gluten, and there's a basic list from www. glutenfreeliving.com). The first 4 weeks, stick with gluten-free grains (quinoa, amaranth, buckwheat, chia, hemp, and flax seeds).

After the first 4 weeks, try the sprouted bread or long-fermented freshly baked breads for toast or sandwiches, steel-cut oats for breakfast, and other grains with gluten in them. But, no white or whole wheat bread conventionally made with modern dwarf wheat, no pasta, and no processed foods that have wheat in them. Stick to whole, intact, unprocessed grains, and the sprouted, long-fermented bread. Observe how you react to gluten. Are you bloated, constipated, congested, gassy, tired, and/or unable to focus? If you feel any of these symptoms, drop wheat and gluten from your diet for good. It's an allergen for you. And you don't need anything inflammatory in your diet.

Here's Aaron E. Carroll's, a Professor of Pediatrics at Indiana University School of Medicine, advice, from a column of his in *The New York Times* on how to eat right: "Get as much of your nutrition as possible from a variety of completely unprocessed foods. These include fruits and vegetables. But they also include meat, fish, poultry and eggs that haven't been processed. In other words, when buying food at the market, focus on things that have not been cooked, prepared or altered in any way. Brown rice over white rice. Whole grains over refined grains. You're far better off eating two apples than drinking the same 27 grams of sugar in an eight-ounce glass of apple juice." And, cook your own food. I know this isn't always easy. It requires time and patience but you can change your habits. All it takes is desire, repetition, and practice. For the first 7 days, you'll definitely want to cook at home. And, after that, when you do go out pick restaurants you know cook food using unprocessed foods—fresh vegetables, whole grains, pasture-raised meat, find places that follow Dr. Carroll's rule of nutrition.

If you're concerned that I've taken away all the food you love, don't be, what you are gaining is a multitude of irresistible, palate and soul satisfying foods to eat. You'll never miss the sugar, dairy, and wheat you're dropping. I know firsthand, as a former sugar, cheese, and bread addict this is 100 percent true. I was the worst when it came to sweets, snacks, low-fat dairy, and fast food. Going back to my roots, the good food I grew up on, I remembered what I forgot, how really delicious whole foods can be. And, to my great delight, I remembered that I enjoy cooking for myself. I used to be the typical New Yorker. It was all prepared foods all the time, and every meal that wasn't a purchased prepared meal from a store was eaten out. I love food, and I love to eat—quantity and quality! And now, I'm happy to be back in the kitchen; it's liberating. What I eat, what I cook, tastes good, and there's never a need to turn to junk food. I have a few friends who tell me: "I don't like cooking for just me." Or, "I don't like to eat what I cook." Well, I love cooking for one. I tailor what I make to my tastes. If I'm in love with a particular dish, like broccoli and edamame salad with avocado dressed simply with lemon juice and olive oil, I can have it every night, and no one will complain about the monotony. And, more than anything I love to eat what I cook. My food tastes best to me. I cook for my tastes, and you need to cook for yours. It's your life, your palate, and your food. Cook what tastes great for you, and I bet most of your family will enjoy what you make.

I promise you this: you will never go hungry on the Ageless Diet, and you will never feel jittery from lack of food. The food you eat will be good enough that you won't miss the bagel, cream cheese, sausage pizza, chocolate cake, pumpkin spice latte, fast food meal deals, or anything else you "treat" yourself to throughout the day. Think about that for a second, the industrial food complex has done such a collective brainwashing on all of us with their ever-present constant advertising that most of us ACTIVELY CHOOSE FOODS THAT ARE UNHEALTHY AS A REWARD. We purposely choose foods that are at best unhealthy and at worst seriously toxic. No big surprise that we as a big, growing nation struggle with weight gain, disease, premature aging, emotional apathy, depression, and general malaise. In order to thrive we must take back control of our diet and our lives and change what "treat yourself" means. Let a reward for a hard day be extra time to meditate, a massage, or a longer walk in the park.

The best thing about quitting all inflammatory foods is that you will stop craving them after the first week. You retrain your palate to want what truly nourishes you. Trust me. I have eaten the wrong way, and now that I'm living for an ageless me, I would never, ever go back. It's not worth it, and the foods I used to eat taste off to me now. They taste overly sweet and salty. They taste like the chemicals used to make them. Of course, if I were in Italy now I would want to taste all the local foods, a little pecorino, prosciutto, pasta, pizza, etc. And that's all right, every now and again, especially when traveling abroad to fabulous food-centric places. But, in general, it's much easier to quit these inflammatory foods altogether. Trying to eat only a moderate amount of dairy, sugar, or wheat keeps me addicted.

Luckily, there are so many really amazing foods I can and do eat.

Even in Italy it would be easy to stay ageless, I could skip the pasta and pizza, eat the farro and grilled vegetables dressed with aged balsamic vinegar and local, cold-pressed olive oil instead. I could forgo the prosciutto and enjoy the fresh fish. The Ageless Diet is really simple. It's about adding a lot of vegetables, fruits, certain types of proteins, and subtracting inflammatory foods.

Our standard, conventional diet leads to toxic overload. And it prevents us from repairing the damage done to our DNA.

DNA is damaged constantly; it's also being repaired constantly. But if you don't have the right raw materials—good diet and lifestyle—you can't repair the damage done, and once the cell divides the damage becomes permanent. Thanks to the targeted support from certain vitamin and mineral supplements we take while on the Ageless Diet, we have help in sustaining and repairing the DNA.

Becoming ageless is as easy as following the **4 Rules**:

1. **Eat Clean.** Anti-inflammatory foods, an organic, mostly plant-based diet. **Drop sugar, dairy, wheat, and all processed foods.** Take vitamin and mineral supplements to augment your diet.

2. **Meditate.** Daily, at least 12 minutes a day.

3. **Exercise.** At least 30 minutes a day, take a walk, practice yoga, work out, etc.

4. **Sleep.** Sleep 7-9 hours a night, with the help of targeted serotonin support supplements.

CHAPTER 28

BOOZE, COFFEE &
THE AGELESS DIET

"Either give me more wine or leave me alone."
—RUMI

A quick note about drinking alcohol on the Ageless Diet: after the *7-Day Cleanse*, alcohol in moderation, meaning a drink or two in the evening, is an option for you.

I like to drink. I love wine, and I love beer. I love the culture of wine, the language of wine, the tastes of different wines from around the world. And, I really enjoy a cold beer. I don't suffer from gluten intolerance, so I can handle a couple of organic, if possible, dark beers in an evening. I especially like pale ales and porters. So, if you're like me, and you really enjoy a glass of wine with dinner then, please, savor it as part of relaxing evening. Enjoy your wine or beer with a delicious, wholesome meal. And if you can handle a little gluten in your diet, explore dark (organic) beers from microbreweries in your area. Obviously, wait till after the first 28 days on the *Reset* to sample beer. Have fun exploring the world of wine; look for wines growing on biodynamic or organic farms. Discover a wine you love from a region you want to visit someday. I had an amazing time in South Africa's Winelands savoring their wines, and eating fabulously fresh foods. Let your love of wine dictate your travel, it's great fun. When you do drink, really enjoy those first sips of the wine, roll it around in your mouth. Notice what flavors or notes you can discover. Make drinking wine a pleasurable part of cooking and unwinding after a day of work, exercise, chores, and running errands. In fact, I almost always cook with wine. I drink wine while I cook!

Obviously, telling you about the health benefits of beer and wine is not advocating drinking or encouraging those of you who prefer opting out of a nightly glass of wine to start consuming alcohol. If you are a non-drinker or can't drink because of health reasons, no need to start now. You're better off without it, if it's not your thing. I just happen to enjoy drinking, so I really savor my nightly wine or beer knowing there are a few ageless benefits that come with moderate drinking. So, without further ado, here are some of those benefits.

> *"I want a beer. I want a giant, ice-cold bottle of beer and shower sex."*
>
> —NORA ROBERTS wrote in *Chasing Fire*

Let's begin with beer. Sometimes just the thing you want on a hot summer day. You'll want to limit your consumption of beer to two, because after two beers any health benefits are outweighed with the detrimental effects of alcohol consumption. Dark beer can be good if you're breastfeeding, but check with your doctor before chugging a cold one. Beer is high in silicon, which is linked to bone health. Pale ales are especially good for bone building. Happily for someone like me who enjoys a frosty beverage, there have been more than 100 studies that show moderate drinking helps limit the risk of heart attacks and dying from cardiovascular disease by 25-40 percent (Harvard University reports). And, one or two micro-brewed beers, like a pale ale, porter, stout, or amber, a day can help raise levels of HDL, the good kind of cholesterol that aids in keeping arteries from clogging. For men, drinking beer can help limit, by 40 percent, the risk of developing kidney stones. *The New England Journal of Medicine* did a study in 2005 that found that a daily beer lowers the risk of mental decline in women and may help prevent Alzheimer's by 20 percent. There was a Dutch study performed at the TNO Nutrition and Food Research Institute that found beer-drinking participants had 30 percent higher levels of vitamin B6 in their blood than their non-drinking friends. Beer also contains vitamin B12 and folic acid. All good news for those of us moderate beer drinkers.

Enough about beer, what about wine, you oenophiles may ask?

> *"Beer is made by men, wine by God."*
> —MARTIN LUTHER

Well, wine is wonderful. Drinking wine can be one of the deep pleasures in life. A glass of vino in the evening can be just what you need to chillax, wind down, and start cooking some beautiful food. Wine drinking promotes longevity—hello, ageless! Wine drinking is good for the heart. It lowers the risk of heart attacks. "Moderate drinkers suffering from high blood pressure are 30 percent less likely to have a heart attack than nondrinkers." (From a 16-year Harvard School of Public Health study of 11,711 men, published in the *Annals of Internal Medicine*, 2007.) I think this happens in part because a glass of wine relaxes the muscles and helps people release tension. And wine drinking lowers the risk of heart disease, type 2 diabetes, colon cancer, and cuts the risk of cataracts. Wine drinking slows brain decline. A study done at Columbia University demonstrated that brain function declines at a markedly faster rate in non-drinkers than in moderate drinkers.

If you are drinking wine, look for organic or biodynamic wines, and stick with mostly red wines. Spend a little more—$10 or $15 for a bottle of wine you'll really enjoy is worth it. Think of the money you're saving by not buying all that processed food and drink, *and* by consuming alcohol more judiciously. It's getting easier and easier to find organic wines that are sulfite free. There's even an unfiltered, organic dry Lambrusco I've fallen in love with that is less than $20. It's divine, and it's lower in alcohol than those big wines—cabs, zins, and syrahs.

Most of us know what organic means, but what does a biodynamic wine mean? Ray Isle in *Food & Wine* explains it this way: "Biodynamic approach to grape-growing sees the vineyard as an ecological whole: not just rows of grapevines, but the soil beneath them—an organism in its own right—and the other flora and fauna in the area, growing together interdependently." I find that the biodynamic and organic wines and beer I drink are easier on my body. There is less chance of suffering from congestion—no sulfites!—or sinus headaches. And the more we support winemakers and brewers who use organic grapes and hops, the more affordable and available these wines and beer become.

Besides enjoying the taste of wine and beer, I like how it forces me to slow down and relax. The English have tea time, and the American south has cultivated a reverence for cocktail hour. I loved how my grandparents, Mitzi and Jimdad, came together at around 5 or 6:00 p.m. for a drink and a review of the day. They relaxed, connected with each other, and fed me snacks. Of course they were cocktail drinkers, not wine lovers, and their snacks were usually crackers and cheese and Chex Mix. But we're not looking to duplicate their drinks and snacks, just the vibe. They had a wonderful, lusty marriage, full of love and fun, and I've got to think strictly observing cocktail hour helped with that. The ritual was the celebration of the end of the work day. The very action of putting work away with a physical bookend and relaxing into the evening is both mentally and physically beneficial.

My recommendation for sticking with beer and wine comes in part because both undergo fermentation, versus the distillation process used to make the harder alcohols, like vodka, rum, whiskey, and scotch. The hard liquor that's best, and in serious moderation, on the Ageless Diet is 100 percent agave made tequila. Studies show this liquor has the fewest impurities. So, if you want a drink and can't have beer or wine, tequila with fresh lime (no more than two) is fine on occasion.

Sometimes with that first sip of wine I can actually feel my muscles release the tension they've been holding onto all day. And once my muscles release, my mind relaxes, and that's a lovely feeling. Suddenly the evening seems full of promise. The prospect of a well-prepared, flavorful meal and engaging conversation at dinner, or the time and space to read a piece in my favorite magazine, if I'm dining solo. And I'm in a frame of mind to really taste my food, to be present to the experience of eating. It's magical. I start to notice the music playing, and I'm more appreciative of the sensuality in preparing and cooking food. It's a fine way to celebrate life and another day on the books. And after supper, I'm happily washing dishes, ready to watch a little TV or read a book and go to sleep soon. Obviously, you don't need a glass of wine or beer to feel this way or to appreciate your life and the food you're eating. I just wanted to let you know that on the Ageless Diet a glass of wine or a beer here and there is totally cool. Or, to paraphrase Lloyd Christmas from the movie *Dumb and Dumber*, let the beer flow like wine.

> *"I'd rather take coffee than compliments just now."*
> —LOUISA MAY ALCOTT in *Little Women*

Coffee is another thing people are unsure about. "Do I have to give up my coffee? Can I still drink my afternoon espresso? Or my pumpkin spice chai latte?" No, no, and no. After the *7-Day Cleanse*, coffee drinking is fine. (If you're dying for caffeine turn to green tea. Matcha is best; it's super green and has a nice strong flavor.) I love coffee like I love wine. I love the smell of it; I love to make it. I like to buy the oily, black beans, and stick my nose in the bag, savoring the strong aroma. I love walking past a boutique coffee shop, inhaling the smell of roasting coffee. I actually like listening to conversations about the origins of the beans, and the best way to prepare it, and why Stumptown makes the best coffee or Blue Bottle or whatever coffee roaster is hot right now. There are people out there who are very passionate about coffee, and I'm into passion. And if you aren't a coffee drinker, if you prefer tea, lucky you. Keep on that train, enjoy a cup of your favorite organic green tea with a little lemon (maximizes the antioxidant benefits of green tea); the vitamin C in lemon juice helps increase the bioavailability of green tea's nutrients.

If you're like me, and you dig coffee, here's how and when you want to consume it. First of all, if you value your sleep, and I know you do because you're on the Ageless Diet, do not drink a caffeinated beverage after 2:00 p.m., stopping by noon would be even better. Drinking coffee late in the day will affect your sleep. And sleep is a beautiful, necessary thing; you want to sleep. It's how you stay ageless. Try to limit yourself to 2 cups a day. No more.

The interesting side effect of eating ageless, and taking supplements, is that most people notice a substantial increase in the level of awareness and overall energy throughout the day. Once those who drink 3-5 cups of coffee a day notice that their previous energy dips and low points in the day have been replaced by higher, more sustained energy levels, limiting their caffeine intake will cease to be an issue. You will feel energized, not wired, and most Ageless Dieters report not needing that jolt of caffeine in the afternoon. When you do drink coffee, try and use only organic, free trade coffee. Coffee beans absorb a helluva lot of pesticides, and you don't need that in your body. Buy the darkest, oiliest beans you can find. The coffee will taste richer than coffee made from dry beans. An oily bean is a sign of freshness, and coffee, like every other organic matter, oxidizes and goes stale. Freshness counts. Grind your own beans and make a ritual out of your coffee drinking if that's your thing, you'll be less prone to head over to the multi-national big box coffee shop and drink a huge burnt offering of a coffee. You'll save money too! Use filtered water. Try a French press. It's easy to use, they are affordable and last forever. Another option is to make an espresso, add extra hot water if you want a big cup of coffee. Lastly, skip the dairy, the sweetener; you don't need it. If you're using really good beans and preparing it well, your coffee will have its own richness, its own natural crema. If you want a little sweetness, try cinnamon. And if you need a cream, try organic coconut, almond, or other plant-based "milk." But first, sample it sans milk of any kind. Just try it . . . isn't that good?

CHAPTER 29

WHY WE SUPPLEMENT

"Millions of Americans today are taking dietary supplements,
practicing yoga and integrating other natural therapies into
their lives. These are all preventive measures that will keep
them out of the doctor's office and drive down the costs of
treating serious problems like heart disease and diabetes."

—ANDREW WEILL

Your map to agelessness is super simple. *Cleanse, Reset,* and follow
the **4 Ageless Rules**: eat vibrant, healthy foods, *supported by vita-*
min, mineral, and herbal supplements, exercise, meditate, and sleep
at least 7 hours a night.

The supplements listed on our program are a great way to help
regulate your sleep, mood, and energy levels throughout the day.
They also make kicking the three bad boys—dairy, sugar, and
wheat—much easier while amplifying the positive effects of this
lifestyle.

Why take supplements? Food is medicine, right? It is, but only
up to a point. I wish things were different. But, they aren't. And, we
won't get ALL the nutrients we need from our food, these days, for
optimal good health. Conventional food comes with extra toxins,
hormones, inflammatory drivers and free radicals that can be too
much for our bodies to manage. We feel better if we supplement
with key core nutrients that support our general health and help
our bodies manage all the unwanted "extras." As Lauren Basso, nutritionist and certified holistic health coach, puts it: "Regardless of

how healthy and balanced our diet is, supplements are essential for everyone. Our soil, food system, and environment are contaminated, and do not provide all the nutrients we need for optimal health. Not to mention, that some of the chemicals, toxins, chronic stress and lack of sleep we all experience on a daily basis, rob us of nutrients, increasing our need that much more, which ultimately cannot be reached by diet alone."

Mineral depletion in soil and in plants, long transit times for food, and loss of natural nutrients cause vitamin and mineral deficiency in foods, meaning we're often deficient in vital nutrients. This loss of nutrients in food means most of us need supplements. "You can trace every sickness, every disease, and every ailment to a mineral deficiency," said Nobel Prize winning chemist, biochemist, peace activist, author, and educator, Linus Pauling.

There are serious toxins in our water supplies, soil—the Earth— is corrupted, and clean air doesn't really exist. Because of industrial farming for the past 50 years or so, soil has been stripped of mineral content. Minerals that plants absorb. The minerals we need are no longer so plentiful in the plants we eat. Add to the mineral depletion in soil, the way we shop for our food and where that food comes from, and we've got serious problems.

We're not often eating food grown out in the backyard. Usually we go to a big grocery store and buy food shipped from far, far away. The long transit times contribute to food that is less fresh and less nutrient-rich. These days the apples I see in the store are from New Zealand. The butternut squash is from Mexico, and the kale is from California. This can mean that by the time the food gets to our local stores, it's far from ideal, in terms of taste and available nutrients. The older the produce, the less nutritional value this produce has. Long transit times mean our apples and berries, our broccoli, are old and not as capable of providing us with the essential vitamins and minerals our bodies require. We sometimes make fun of the rabid locavores and their insistence on all food being locally sourced, but they're right. They do have a powerful point. The more food we buy locally and in season, the more we'll have access to, and the more nutrient-rich that food will be. Here's my quick Public Service Announcement: shop local, shop organic. As they say, pay your farmer not your doctor. Eat whole (intact) grains, organic fruits, vegetables, legumes, nuts, and seeds, pasture-raised meats and eggs, and drink filtered water.

Most people are chronically deficient in at least several essential nutrients. This is a disaster for our health. Chronic deficiency of even one essential nutrient causes disease and accelerates aging. The modern diet is so bad (and nutrient deficient) that Dr. Carl Pfeiffer, author of *Mental and Elemental Nutrients*, writes that, "The average human diet, nutritionally unfit for rats, must be equally unsatisfactory or even more so in meeting human needs." The National Academy of Sciences issued a report in 1997, when the water, air, and soil were a little less polluted than they are now, stating it is no longer possible to get all the nutrition (from food) needed for optimal health.

Currently greenhouse gases are also causing lower nutrients in food. Rising carbon dioxide levels drain crops of life-saving nutrients. Samuel Myers, MD, MPH, research scientist in the department of environmental health at Harvard School of Public Health and lead author in a landmark study on this subject, said the loss of nutrients in food is "an enormous public health problem today."

Excessive toxins absorbed from our environments lead to inflammation and disease, and premature aging. The ongoing loss of minerals in the soil, and the widespread use of pesticides, preservatives, and chemicals to grow, harvest, and transport food means greater toxicity. To get well and stay well we must lessen the ill effects of that toxic overload. Supplements, in conjunction with a clean diet, can help us deal with these "extras"—pollutants, toxins, and stresses—we come in contact with on a daily basis. They can be useful in restoring us to good health and a place of balance.

I've learned from research and experiential evidence that supplements work, enhancing the positive changes made in diet and lifestyle. They help repair and revitalize the immune system and metabolism. But, I understand the critics' arguments against drugstore vitamins and minerals. Lesser supplements are often unregulated or made in poorly regulated manufacturing facilities with token doses, and cheaper, less bioavailable forms of nutrients and herbs or herbal extracts. Because it's hard to find high quality supplements and to know which ones to take, I make it easy for you. In this book I list the supplements key for ageless living, explain why they are a necessity, and on AgelessDietLife.com our team of nutritionists, naturopathic doctors, and wellness experts source them for you. If you are unsure about supplements, consult your own doctor, a nutritionist, or an Ageless Diet expert listed on our site about what is right for you.

According to Carrie Daenell, ND, a leading practitioner and nutritional supplement expert, "Most nutritional supplements on the market are so close and yet so far away from being what you hope they are. Seeking credible guidance when making nutritional supplement selections is like gaining trusted advice when choosing a mechanic, a surgeon or an accountant—taking care to make smart choices makes all the difference in the care you are taking of yourself."

Before I tried our supplement program, I always believed that a diet of kale smoothies, anti-inflammatory meals, and a modest amount of dark chocolate and red wine, was enough. I was the one who always, *always*, told people, you don't need supplements if you're eating right—get everything you need from the produce section of your grocery store. Boy, was I wrong. The right supplements can help you feel better, get healthy, and cool down inflammation.

I wanted to discover for myself whether supplementation really works. When I committed to a comprehensive supplement program I went all in. By all in I mean *all in,* the one I tested first was comprised of dozens of supplements, taken daily. It seemed excessive and ridiculous. I felt the hit in my wallet. I actively hoped they wouldn't work because the first supplement program was expensive, but mostly because I loved being right. Kale smoothies are all the vitamins you need! Well, I was wrong. Within a week I felt dramatically better. Actually, within two days, I had more energy throughout the day, a cleaner energy, with fewer dips, and I slept better. That first week I had to stop drinking coffee and take extra walks around the block, I was so energized.

Three days into my first week taking supplements I felt good. I was revitalized. (Of course, I was also eating better than I had in over 20 years.) I went to an integrative health conference in Dallas, and I worked the conference. That meant 18 hours a day for 4 full days. And my conference partner, Blair, was eating Ageless Diet style for those 4 days but he wasn't taking the supplements, and he was dragging. He wasn't sleeping the few hours a night we got, and he was tired during the day. I felt good. I felt better than anyone else at the conference. I looked better too. These conferences are marathons of work and schmoozing. And, I was forced to admit, supplements made the difference. Not to overstate it, but they were a game changer. They changed my mind and the Ageless Diet forevermore. And, while I was hustling at the conference, Scott was at home taking the same supplements. He felt better too. He couldn't believe it. No lethargy in the afternoon, aches and pains were less prevalent, and he had more energy for his workouts, for work, and for life in general. After those first 2 weeks, we jumped on the supplement train and never got off. And I've never regretted it. In fact, it's made a huge difference in every part of my life. Of course, these positive effects from targeted supplement support wouldn't have been possible—or even felt—if we hadn't already been eating clean and exercising regularly. If you're eating trash, living a sedentary lifestyle, first fix your lifestyle, clean up your diet, otherwise it is lipstick on a pig; the supplements are wasted.

Blair, who wasn't yet supplementing his diet with vitamins and minerals, was still exhausted for weeks after the conference. Blair, like many of us, sometimes suffers from depression and bouts of insomnia. He finally succumbed to my hectoring and lecturing, started to eat clean and exercise regularly, and he went on a field trip with me for supplements, mostly to shut me up. But it worked. He changed his diet and lifestyle, and he took the supplements. Within a few days he was feeling brighter, more focused, and his mood lifted. It's not always a dramatic uplift, but it's one you can definitely feel. Blair quits the program every now and again but he always comes back to it, after he gets tired of feeling low.

Scott noticed that when he started taking omega-3s he stopped the pain medication he routinely availed himself of during a regular work day. Most daily aches and pains disappeared. Omega-3s are very anti-inflammatory (so much so that when I had a special kind of intense facial in South Africa they told me to stop taking them because the inflammation on my face was what they wanted to stimulate collagen growth).

Since I've been on the program I've traveled to South Africa—a 37 hour trip sans sleep—and back several times for projects, with little to no jet lag. None. This is a blessing. Because, did you know jet lag causes weight gain? "Thanks to our own rhythms, we eat at regular times of the day, and it's these feeding patterns that drive the cycles in our microbiome. Diet is the gear that synchronises the ticks of our clocks with those of our microbes," explains Ed Yong in a piece for the *National Geographic*. Jet lag messes with our natural rhythms, including those of our very important microbiome. (The gut! Good health always goes back to the gut.) Sticking with an Ageless Diet on the road, taking probiotics, combined with the added support from the supplement program, can mitigate the negative effects long distance travel has on the body.

Scott found jet-lag-free travel to be some kind of crazy miracle. Before South Africa, the last time he flew on a very long trip was several years ago. He went to China, and on his return he was wiped out. He was unable to focus or sleep at night for more than a few hours, and he collapsed in the afternoon every day for over a week. This year's trip to South Africa was a longer flight than the one to China, and there was no jet lag, there and back. Of course, he was eating ageless this time. This supplement program working in conjunction with an anti-inflammatory diet and lifestyle does its job beautifully, giving you extra energy and vitality. It works for you on an average day at home, and supports you on those 37-hour days in the air. Don't leave home without your ageless-approved supplements.

The vitamins and minerals that are part of our ageless toolkit are an easy way to ensure that the body gets a steady supply of essential nutrients.

What do vitamins do for us? It's simple. They accelerate cell repairs, which slows down aging.

CHAPTER 30

AGELESS DIET SUPPLEMENTS

"Vitamins and minerals are the essential nutrients we require daily in order to function normally and efficiently."

This supplement program was created to give you maximum wellness and good health. They work best when taken for longer than the initial 6 weeks. Vitamins are complex molecules required for normal functions in our bodies. Minerals are critical in building the body's cells. Minerals are referred to as the building blocks of the body.

Included in **the Ageless Diet Supplement Program** are the necessary basics: **Omega-3, Vitamin D3, Probiotics, Vitamin B Complex,** a first-rate **Multivitamin,** and the powerhouse anti-inflammatory **Turmeric (optimized curcumin).**

Vitamin D, a.k.a., the "sunshine vitamin," plays many important roles in the proper functioning of the body. Though classified as a vitamin, D is actually a key regulatory hormone for calcium and bone metabolism. Adequate vitamin D status is essential for ensuring normal calcium absorption and maintenance of healthy plasma calcium levels. Besides this essential bone support, vitamin D has many other roles in the body: modulation of cell growth, neuromuscular and immune function and inflammatory support. It's a key vitamin in for cooling down inflammation. Make sure you take the right type of vitamin D. The only active form of vitamin D is vitamin D3 (cholecalciferol). This is the type you want. Many vitamins and prescriptions of vitamin D have vitamin D2—which is not biologically active. And, be sure to take the right amount of vitamin D. If you have a deficiency, you can correct it with 5,000 to 10,000 IU of vitamin D3 a day for 3 months, but only under a doctor's supervision. And, for maintenance, you may take 2,000 to 4,000 IU a day of vitamin D3. Because many scientists now believe that supplementation with vitamin D at higher levels than previously thought necessary is vital to maintaining healthy bone remodeling and healthy vitamin D plasma levels.

Probiotics: the support we need for a healthy gut. I'm obsessed with the health of my gut, with good reason. As you know, post-gut chapter, a healthy gut is essential for optimal wellness. And one easy way to maintain the health of your microbiome is with a high-quality probiotic. What are probiotics? They are oral supplements of live, beneficial intestinal micro-organisms for nutritional health and well-being. Antibiotics tend to kill off both beneficial and harmful bacteria, and disturb the normal, healthy balance of intestinal microorganisms. Toxins absorbed in the environment and from our food also disrupt the healthy balance of beneficial bacteria in our gut. Various intestinal conditions can compromise the immune system and lower the amounts of healthy intestinal microflora. Probiotics exert beneficial support of the immune system through changes or modifications to the gut environment. The health of the gut affects the health of the immune system. Bifido-bacterium lactis HN019 (found in many of the better, higher-grade probiotics) has been clinically shown in research to support the immune system by enhancing the function of leucocytes in adults and the elderly. This strain may also help in the maintenance of bowel regularity and normal GI function. Dr. Daenell—a go-to digestive repair doctor in Naturopathic Medicine—says, from experience: "The gut is like Mama—if it ain't happy, nothing is healthy." She goes on to say, "Probiotics are something we would all do well to supplement in today's world. They support immune function, nutrient absorption, healthy cholesterol levels and reduce risk for many of the diseases of aging." Be sure to source a probiotic that actually works, check AgelessDietLife.com for help with this.

Omega-3 fatty acids are polyunsaturated fatty acids and essential nutrients for optimal health. An omega-3 supplement is one of the most important on the list. You want to make sure you're getting 3000 mg (3 grams) of omega-3s every day, and more if you're dealing with serious chronic inflammation.

Everyone knows by now that omega-3s are necessary for good health, but why? Short answer: omega-3s are a really effective anti-inflammatory. They aid in cooling down inflammation, and they are the one supplement you definitely want to spend the extra money on, to ensure you're taking a high-grade one that actually works.

What will omega-3s do for you? Help with dry skin. They are a necessity for maintaining healthy and supple skin. Omega-3s repair the protective barrier that keeps moisture locked in. Combining an omega-3 supplement with regular exercise has been shown to improve cardiovascular and metabolic health. They reduce the risk of heart disease.

Ms. Basso, nutritionist, health coach, and Ageless Diet consultant, says this about the top three essentials in a basic supplement program:

> We all need to utilize supplements if we want vibrant health. Much of the recommended daily intake (RDI) for vitamins and minerals is set at the bare minimum to avoid deficiencies. However, these levels are still suboptimal. We need to take *additional* steps to ensure we are meeting and exceeding our daily micronutrient requirements. Almost all of us benefit from taking an omega-3 fish oil, a probiotic, and a vitamin D, at the minimum, not to mention a high-quality multivitamin. All these micronutrients are hard to get from food alone. And lifestyle behaviors, including diet, deplete these nutrients. They all have a profound impact on our health and wellness.
>
> Firstly, omega-3 is essential to our bodies. With so much of our food system plagued with omega-6 oils, which is also essential to our bodies, though in smaller doses than most currently eat, it is challenging to get enough omega-3 fat. The problem with the modern diet is that the ratio of omega-3 to omega-6 is dramatically out of balance, causing widespread inflammation,

affecting everything from cognitive health to joints. Supplementing with omega-3 ensures this ratio is more balanced, and it keeps inflammation at bay. Probiotics are another big hitter. Our entire body is comprised of billions of tiny organisms that play critical functions, especially in supporting our gastrointestinal health. GI health influences not just our immune system but neurological function, hormone production, and detoxification as well. Therefore, if our gut bacteria are out of balance, which can easily happen with poor diet (too much sugar, caffeine, alcohol), use of antibiotics, chronic stress, or exposure to chemicals, we're out of balance. Needless to say, even if your diet is well balanced, you cannot escape the other factors that influence your bacterial balance, thus probiotics provide a good safety net for everyone. Lastly, vitamin D is so impactful on our health. We're seeing epidemic levels of suboptimal vitamin D. It's so important to know what your vitamin D levels are and supplement accordingly. Vitamin D is crucial to every single cell in our bodies, therefore this small little hormone has a big effect on bone and immune health, hormone balance, and gene expression. [Note: if you want more information on having your vitamin D levels, among others, checked, go to our site, and we'll point you in the right direction.]

A really good, comprehensive multivitamin can help fill in the gaps. Studies have shown we all need a basic high-quality, broad-spectrum multivitamin and mineral. Micronutrient supplementation, like those found in the type of multivitamin we recommend on AgelessDietLife.com, can help alleviate symptoms from mental and physical illnesses.

In addition to a multivitamin, a D3, a probiotic, and an omega-3, I'm a big fan a good vitamin B complex. It keeps me feeling energized. The eight B vitamins—B1, B2, B3, B5, B6, B7, B9, B12—play important roles in keeping our bodies strong and healthy. These nutrients help convert our food into fuel, energizing us all day. They are essential and central in cellular metabolism (the metabolism of lipids, carbohydrates, and proteins). The majority of these B vitamins are coenzymes for many important enzymes involved in anabolic and catabolic reactions. They are important for blood cells, hormones, and nervous system function. As water-soluble substances, B vitamins are not stored in the body in any appreciable amounts, so we need an adequate supply of B vitamins on a daily basis. They work in tandem, and each has its own specific benefit. We've included a powerful B-complex with folate (or folic acid), B6, and B12 on the supplement program because they are energy boosters. As co-enzymes, the B vitamins are essential components in most major metabolic reactions. B vitamins work together synergistically, so look for a quality supplement with all the Bs. You'll want one that contains methylcobalamin, a coenzyme form of B12, because studies indicate it may be better utilized and better retained in the body.

I wanted an optimized **curcumin** or **turmeric** supplement on our list because it's a powerful anti-inflammatory. We're all about cooling down inflammation. And, besides taking a supplement with optimized curcumin, I highly recommend cooking with turmeric as much as possible; it's a gorgeous spice to use in a variety of dishes. The active curcuminoids in turmeric help protect against the oxidative stress that accelerates premature skin aging. A good curcumin supplement will contain a high level of all the main active curcuminoids in turmeric. This spice is renowned for its anti-inflammatory effects, and it is proven to help with accelerated wound healing, colon and gallbladder health, improved mental and brain function, anti-aging, and maintaining normal blood sugar levels. Find the best quality curcumin supplement you can and cook with turmeric as often as you can.

For added energy, included on the program are a group of supplements that protect the mitochondria against free radical damage, support cellular energy production, and stimulate phospholid synthesis. Scientific ways of saying these guys are big deals on the anti-aging front. They'll also give your metabolism a jumpstart. They are **L-Carnosine, CoQ10, Acetyl-L-Carnitine,** and **Alpha Lipoic Acid**.

Alpha lipoic acid is found only in trace amounts in food, so we supplement. For healthy skin and body, alpha lipoic acid is one of the more powerful antioxidant supplements available. It can help prevent signs of aging by maintaining a cell's metabolic function for optimal performance. And when it comes to kicking your metabolism into a higher gear, alpha lipoic acid works as a coenzyme in the production of energy by converting carbohydrates into energy.

One of the best amino acids for agelessness is **L-Carnosine.** This supplement is an antioxidant, renowned for specifically targeting anti-aging. I take 500 mg of L-carnosine midday. L-carnosine (or simply carnosine) is a naturally occurring combination of two amino acids. Carnosine was discovered in Russia in the early 1900s. Scientific experiments have shown that carnosine rejuvenates cells, keeping those telomeres long. Cells cultured with carnosine lived longer and retained their youthful appearances and growth patterns. As with all supplements, quality counts. If you walked into your local drugstore and bought a bottle of carnosine, you wouldn't have much luck finding one that does what it promises. Much of the carnosine out there is very low-grade. In fact, it's useless. One big reason the low-grade stuff is used is that carnosine isn't cheap. And most companies simply use one that's neither useful nor bioavailable. The effectiveness builds gradually. Take it every day for this anti-aging powerhouse to do its job.

Acetyl-L-carnitine is also part of the ageless program. Acetyl-L-carnitine improves mitochondrial function. (Mitochondria is the power plant of your cells.) It's an amino acid that works as an energizer. Acetyl-L-carnitine can be important for weight loss because it acts as a natural anti-inflammatory. It also enhances the sensitivity of insulin receptors, helping to decrease blood sugar and circulating levels of insulin. High levels of insulin are inflammatory and lead to premature aging and weight gain. It's also good for improved cognitive functions. Acetyl-L-carnitine is the carnitine form that can reach the brain. There have been many clinical studies showing that this added energy boost slows down Alzheimer's disease and other forms of dementia. As demonstrated by many well-designed scientific studies, carnitine plays a key role in maintaining normal brain and nerve function during aging. It has also been shown to maintain cellular membrane stability and restore the cell membrane to ageless.

Coenzyme Q10 or CoQ10 is an ageless-approved supplement because it's a powerful antioxidant/anti-inflammatory. It can help prevent obesity. Like acetyl-L-carnitine, CoQ10 assists in energy production within the mitochondria. Because energy production declines as a cell ages, the cell's ability to repair itself also declines, which is where CoQ10 comes in handy. Working with acetyl-l-carnitine and alpha lipoic acid in the mitochondria, CoQ10 boosts the metabolism and gives us greater energy and more endurance. It helps with weight loss by maximizing the burning of foods for fuel. CoQ10 assists in preventing the energy decline seen in aging cells. I take 100 mg of CoQ10 daily. CoQ10 is found in small amounts in food like sardines, salmon, and nuts, but for serious ageless benefits and help with weight loss supplementation is a good thing.

For that extra support I use a naturally flavored, rather tasty vegetarian protein powder in my detox smoothies during the *Reset*. I also add it to smoothies when I'm very busy with work and meetings, or on set all day, and may be skipping meals. It's especially useful on the *Cleanse* portion of the *Reset*. My favorite protein powder is a combination of rice and pea proteins. It is also supports the *Cleanse* with essential amounts of vitamins, minerals, antioxidants and other nutrients important for the healthy maintenance of the entire gastrointestinal tract. It's designed to be a complete gastrointestinal support formula, perfect for detoxification. If you want to use my favorite protein powder, check the site, or if sourcing your own, please make sure it contains no artificial colors or preservatives and is lactose, gluten, heavy metal and pesticide-free.

For mood support and help with sleep, try a prolonged release **Melatonin, L-Theanine, GABA (gamma amino butyric acid),** and **Passion Flower Extract.** They are known to help to calm the brain, ease nervous energy, and lessen anxiety. And melatonin can help make quality sleep a possibility for those sleep-challenged.

I'm not saying that supplements are miracle pills or cure-alls, but in conjunction with a clean diet they support an ageless you. Supplements can give you energy, jumpstart your day, help you sleep, detoxify, and cool down inflammation. As Ms. Basso, our nutritionist and health coach, says, "Inflammation, without question is one of the major underlying factors of almost every major disease. This includes anything from premature aging, obesity, heart disease, high blood pressure to arthritis. Chronic inflammation is the leading culprit."

The Ageless Diet Supplement Program was created because all of these parts put together work. It was as simple as that. And with the guidance of respected naturopathic doctors and nutritionists, we have sourced the highest quality supplements to give you the best support. The focus is on the quality of raw materials, the manufacturing process, quality control testing, and therapeutic dose. Our program includes vitamins and minerals selected for optimal, ageless living from a pure, reliable source. If you source your own supplements, please find the best you can. Here's Ms. Basso on that: "Not all supplements are created equally. The biggest differences between a product you'll find on the shelves at your local supplement shop and something your healthcare practitioner is selling are quality and label verification, meaning what is stated on the label is actually in the product." And, of course, for more information and recommendations on supplements, go to AgelessDietLife.com

Ageless Diet Supplement Program

1. **Multivitamin,** a.m./p.m. (follow the recommended dosage, taking 1-3 daily)

2. **Omega-3,** a.m. (or a.m./p.m., depending on the recommended dosage), aim for three 1,000 mg with a ratio of EPA/DHA 300/200

3. **B Complex,** once a day (in morning or midday), B6-50 mg, B12-1000 mg with at least half from a methylcobalamin & folate (folic acid) 800 mcg with at least half from the active form or 5-MTHF (l-methylfolate)

4. **Probiotic,** with at least 15 billion organisms, you can go up

to several 100 billion if you want, once a day, in the morning

5. **D3** (in the active form- cholecalciferol) 2,000-5,000 IU, once a day in the AM, with breakfast

6. **Optimized Curcumin** (Turmeric) 100 mg, a strong anti-inflammatory, twice a day, a.m. and p.m.

Energy Support

1. **Co-Enzyme Q10** (ubiquinone), midday

2. **Acetyl-L-Carnitine,** midday

3. **Alpha-Lipoic Acid,** midday

4. **L-Carnosine,** midday

Sleep + Mood Support

1. **GABA** (gamma-aminobutyric acid), 100-500 mg, bedtime

2. **Passion flower** (Passiflora incarnate L.), 100 mg, bedtime

3. **L-Theanine,** 100 mg, bedtime

4. **Melatonin,** 3-6 mg, prolonged release, bedtime

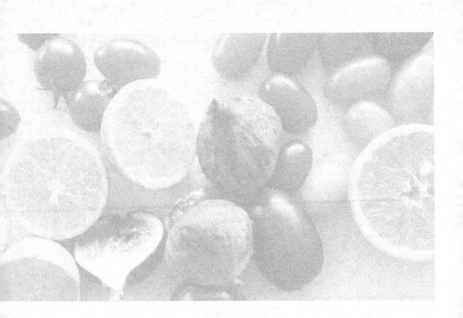

PART 3

Meditate

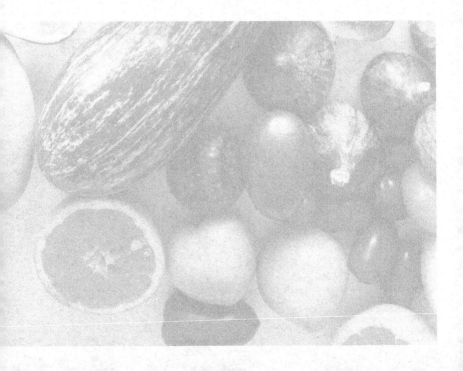

PART 3

Wetlands

CHAPTER 31

MEDITATE YOUR WAY TO A BETTER WORLD

"The more man meditates upon good thoughts,
the better will be his world and the world at large."
—CONFUCIUS

The first rule of the Ageless Diet: Eat Clean. (Drop Sugar, Dairy, and Wheat.) The second rule, Meditate, is even simpler. Carve out 12 minutes of your day and meditate. Embrace the practice of meditation and open the door to a more easeful way of living.

There are few things you can do for yourself that are as effective in cooling down inflammation as meditation. A meditation practice can shift the energy, yours and the world around you. There have been multiple studies done on group meditations that have demonstrated the effects meditation has on outside forces. Pollution levels and crime rates drop, all because of meditation. If we can get that kind of result with a big city, imagine what a daily meditation practice can do for *your* mind, body, and spirit. If a dozen of us, here in New York, meditated on peace the whole city would feel the effects.

Meditation is a practice. Do it every day. If you do, you'll probably end up like me, the least likely person *ever* to meditate, and find yourself craving your daily down time. It will become like sleep to you: necessary and rejuvenating.

A 12-minute daily meditation practice is a game changer. You'll be more productive in your workday and you'll sleep better. You'll make smarter decisions in your day-to-day life. And, even better, you'll become more mindful. You'll find yourself more able to concentrate. It's one of the easiest, cheapest things you can do that will have the biggest, most positive effect on your life. How many things can you say that about?

"Meditation is acceptance. It is the acceptance of life within us, without us and all around us. Acceptance of life is the beginning of human satisfaction. Transformation of life is the culmination of divine satisfaction."
— Sri Chinmoy

What is meditation? A state of thoughtless awareness—you're aware, and thoughts float past you like clouds. It's this state that brings peace and grace. When you're able to drop in and really meditate, even if you're only in that sweet spot for a minute, this process of quieting your mind allows you to tap into the universal flow. You're floating in infinite possibility. You can meditate standing up, in line at the grocery store, waiting for the train, or while gardening. I prefer to do it comfortably seated, with my eyes closed. And for you, I recommend the same. This state of profound peace occurs when the mind is calm and alert. You're tuning in, turning on, and tapping into your own infinite source. If that's too much for you, consider this, you're quieting your mind, calming down, and feeling better. It's a 12-minute practice you can pretty much do anywhere, anytime.

Deepak Chopra says: "Everyone thinks that the purpose of meditation is to handle stress, to tune out, to get away from it all. While that's partially true, the real purpose of meditation is actually to tune in, not to get away from it all, *but to get in touch with it all.* Not to just de-stress, but to find that peace within, the peace that spiritual traditions talk about that passes all understanding." In meditation, we have the opportunity to discover infinite possibilities and to access our own infinite potential. We have the chance to connect with the divine aspect of ourselves. And that's magical.

Even if you're not able to quiet your mind 100 percent, you still reap benefits. I try to meditate every day. I like to do it for an hour. You might gasp, "An hour! I don't have that kind of time." I totally understand; *it's a whole hour.* Who spends an hour on himself, never mind on meditation? Who has an hour to waste? It's not like anyone is watching an hour of TV or mindlessly chasing the next hyperlink online for that long. Oh wait . . . maybe we do spend a lot of time staring at screens for non-work-related reasons.

Build it into your day as you would anything, meals, sleep, work, and exercise. I do. An hour meditation practice works for me because it takes me almost an hour to calm my crazy, busy mind down. I have a mind that won't stop whirring, and my brain is too full sometimes. Often when I meditate, I run through my list of things to do, my list of grievances, and everything else I'm thinking about that day. I know you have a busy brain too, but I hope you're better at chilling out than I am. For me, the first 38 minutes of my meditation are often spent running through facts and figures and gossip. And then, after that is exhausted, I finally breathe, in and out, in and out, letting the thoughts float by me like so many clouds. And, though I am not a natural at this, I do feel better after every meditation, calmer, more focused, and more cheerful. I usually sleep much better on the days I meditate. My busy little brain is one reason people like me often meditate first thing in the morning. My friend and former business partner, Sheila, wakes at 4 :00 a.m. to meditate. I just can't. I have a breakfast, coffee routine I'm attached to, and I like a meditation mid-afternoon. At 2:00 p.m. when my energy dips, I restore the core *me* to me with meditation (followed by a kale smoothie). And, when I don't have a whole hour to meditate, I'll make sure to do a 12-minute one. It makes me feel better. It's not sexy, and it's not expensive, but it works. And, it can help smooth out wrinkles and worries. Meditation is seriously anti-aging.

Meditation keeps you ageless. It activates the **immortality enzyme**. What's that? Remember those telomeres, the ends of DNA strands that get shorter as we age? Well, telomerase acts on the ends of DNA strands. Telomerase, the immortality enzyme, builds the equivalent of caps at the end of DNA shoelaces. Weihang Chai of

Washington State University, who found a way to kill cancer cells by deactivating the enzyme telomerase, which causes them to age and die like normal cells, discovered that if you can turn off the telomerase of cancer cells, perhaps you can find a way to keep the immortality enzyme on in normal cells. If the enzyme keeps building new caps, a DNA strand can replicate indefinitely. Hence, it's immortality. We stop making telomerase as we age, but meditation can help with that.

"Scientists at the University of California at Los Angeles and Nobel Prize winner Elizabeth Blackburn found that 12 minutes of daily yoga meditation for eight weeks increased telomerase activity by 43 percent, suggesting an improvement in stress-induced aging. Blackburn of the University of California, San Francisco, shared the Nobel medicine prize in 2009 with Carol Greider and Jack Szostak for research on the telomerase 'immortality enzyme,' which slows the cellular aging process," writes Makiko Kitamura in *Business Week*.

Isn't it marvelous that something as simple as meditation can turn on the *immortality enzyme*? A daily meditation practice helps the body function on a level that's several years younger than its chronological age. A study published in the *International Journal of Neuroscience* showed subjects, with an average chronological age of 50 years, who had practiced meditation (specifically Transcendental Meditation) for over 5 years, had a biological age 12 years younger than their chronological age. That's pretty significant. That makes 30 the new 20, for real. And if you're 40, well, then you're basically 28. Who cares about chronological age if your biological one is forever young? You'll have it all: experience and vitality!

And the case for meditation gets more compelling. John Denninger, a psychiatrist at Harvard Medical School, is doing a five-year study on how the ancient practices of yoga and meditation affect genes and brain activity in the chronically stressed. This follows a study he and others published that shows how mind-body techniques, meditation and yoga (exercise), can switch on and off some genes linked to stress and immune function. Reaction to stress can lead to inflammation, weight gain, and premature aging.

And, Harvard's study demonstrates meditation cools down aging inflammation from stress.

If you find you consistently live a high stress life—and doesn't everyone these days?—this is especially good news. "Unlike earlier studies, this one is the first to focus on participants with high levels of stress. The study published in May 2014 in the medical journal PLOS One showed that one session of relaxation-response practice was enough to enhance the expression of genes involved in energy metabolism and insulin secretion and reduce expression of genes linked to inflammatory response and stress. There was an effect even among novices who had never practiced before," writes Ms. Kitamura.

Meditation helps shape how you think and directs your mind to more positive thoughts. This is more good news because *what you think and how you think* can decide the level of health you enjoy. It's not mind over matter; it's the mind *does* matter. Our bodies listen to our minds. Want to change the way you feel? Meditate, and your body will respond. In the same way that what you eat affects how you think, what your mind thinks changes how your body feels. Meditation calms your mind, and you respond to aging stressors in a more effective, balanced way. Think about what you think about. Become a more conscious thinker, use meditation as an essential tool in this endeavor.

"Positive psychological changes that occur during meditation. . . . are associated with greater telomerase activity, according to researchers at the University of California, Davis, and the University of California, San Francisco. The study is the first to link positive well-being to higher telomerase, an enzyme important for the long-term health of cells, in the body. The effect appears to be attributable to psychological changes that increase a person's ability to cope with stress and maintain feelings of well-being. 'We have found that meditation promotes positive psychological changes, and that meditators showing the greatest improvement on various psychological measures had the highest levels of telomerase,' said Clifford Saron, associate research scientist at the UC Davis Center for Mind and Brain." (From the University of California, Davis)

Meditation is also amazingly helpful for people with high blood pressure, hypertension, panic attacks, and anxiety attacks. People with autoimmune diseases like lupus, asthma, and other illnesses caused by inflammation benefit greatly from a regular meditation practice. It cools down inflammation.

My life has improved in part thanks to meditation. I'm more creative, or perhaps it's that I'm more productive. It used to be when an idea would float my way, I'd oftentimes just let it sit there, until the creative inspiration disappeared. Now, I have a more thoughtful, mindful approach, which helps me pursue ideas and create something out of them. I believe a lot of this drive to create comes from meditating. And it's made me happier. And, perhaps as useful as drive and focus, meditation is an energizing reboot.

So, what else can meditation do for you? *Help prevent brain disease.* This is a huge one for me, since Mitzi, my grandmother, died of Alzheimer's. It was dreadful watching that disease take over her brain and body and eventually kill her. Alzheimer's is an awful disease. And more and more people are victims of it, which means, as with most diseases prevalent in our society these days, the causes are most likely environmental. (Environmental, meaning what we eat, where we live, how we live.) A 2010 study in the *Journal of Alzheimer's Disease* showed that meditation reduces and possibly reverses the effects of Alzheimer's disease. Practicing meditation 12 minutes a day, for just 8 weeks, increased brain activity in areas important to memory. This daily 12-minute practice was shown to improve cognition and well-being in patients with memory loss.

For those of you who practice yoga regularly, let's not forget the real goal in yoga, which is to loosen the body up enough to keep a steady seat and meditate. In fact, in Ayurvedic medicine, a deep level of relaxation, which meditation brings, is considered necessary before the healing can begin. Isn't that beautiful? To heal, we must relax.

Meditation makes you smarter, and it reduces stress and anxiety levels. Before you hit the Xanax, try meditation. In a study published in an issue of *Psychiatry Research: Neuroimaging*, a meditation practice was found to lead to increases in regional brain gray matter density. M.R.I. brain scans taken before and after the participants' meditation practice discovered increased activity in the gray matter in the hippocampus, an area important for learning and memory. Even better, the images demonstrated a reduction in activity around the gray matter in the amygdala, the region connected to stress and anxiety. The M.R.I. showed that meditation reduces stress and anxiety. Meditation thickens the brain's cortex, and it lowers blood pressure. And, what about the control group that didn't meditate? No changes. So, if you want to relax the part of your brain connected with anxiety, meditate. It's the cheapest, fastest, easiest way to calm your nerves, feel better, and lengthen your telomeres and your life. Wow, that's kind of a miracle.

As you can probably tell by now, there have been many scientific studies on the benefits of meditation. One study suggests that meditation may lower heart attack risk. And, of course, for everyone out there claiming to have Attention Deficit Disorder (more than half my New Yorker friends swear they've got A.D.D.) there have been studies showing the connection between meditation and attention span. As you may have guessed, meditation lengthens your attention span, giving you focus, energy, and the will to move forward with tasks. Meditation could make your A.D.D. a thing of the past, or at the very least manageable.

Be a better person, meditate. There have been several recent studies suggesting that meditation alters structures in the brain. "In a 2008 study published in the journal *PloS One*, researchers found that when meditators heard the sounds of people suffering, they had stronger activation levels in their temporal parietal junctures, a part of the brain tied to empathy, than people who did not meditate," writes Sindya N. Bhanoo in *The New York Times*. Empathy can be used as powerful force for positive social transformation. Through building a more empathetic attitude we can improve the lives of everyone around us, including our own. Cultivating empathy makes us more curious about life, and this increases our satisfaction with our own lives. It's empathy that encourages us to be more generous and more compassionate with others. Practicing kindness and empathy has been shown to make people happier.

One of the easiest ways to feel better is to be of service to someone else. And, if meditation increases the kinder, more empathetic side of your personality, you'll probably find you want to help others, which will likely make you feel better. You meditate, you're more empathetic, you're kinder, then you're happier, and then you meditate more.

Meditation keeps you healthy. There have also been several studies demonstrating a connection between meditation and improved immune function. The University of Wisconsin's study suggests "that meditation, long promoted as a technique to reduce anxiety and stress, might produce important biological effects that improve a person's resiliency." (From *Science Daily*)

Remember, it's the daily meditation practice that really makes the difference in life. It's called a practice for a reason. This means it requires daily practice, because only in the regular routine of meditating do you absorb all the wonderful benefits. It's only 12 minutes a day. We all have room in our lives for 12 minutes, especially if it keeps you healthy and ageless. We've paid a lot more, in time and money, for anti-aging products, haven't we?

I've been meditating for over 4 years now. Sometimes I have a mind blowing, expansive experience, but mostly I don't. And that's ok, because I feel better, more present, and calmer. But I don't always come away from my practice feeling wonder with a deeper insight about the ways of the world. I do feel more relaxed and a greater ease and clarity more often, because meditation has a cumulative effect. I feel less stressed by the daily vagaries of life. I feel refreshed after each meditation. And, I feel more grounded. I'm able to process the stressful events in my life better and more quickly. If I spend an hour meditating, and all I do is focus on my problems, my monkey mind obsessively revisiting whatever is bothering me that day, then it's not a very successful practice. BUT even then I do feel better. And, because I used up my meditation practice that day obsessing over the problem vexing me, the anxiety around it dissipates, almost magically. This is why the daily practice is key. Because some days you'll fly, floating up effortlessly, and other days you're lucky if you're able to focus mindfully for the space of a single breath. Either way, though, you'll feel better by the end of it. AND, you'll definitely feel rejuvenated and restored after just the first few weeks of daily meditation. Big problems will seem manageable, and small, day-to-day stresses inconsequential. If John D. Rockefeller and Thomas Edison swore by their afternoon respite for clarity, improved focus, and daily stress management, why not give it a try. If we're talking about things that age us, let's talk stress.

CHAPTER 32

REFRAME STRESS

*"Always believe that
something wonderful is about to happen."*
—SUKHRAJ S. DHILLON

We deal with stress every day. It ain't going anywhere. The time has come to learn how to successfully manage stress. Here's what stress does to our bodies (and our minds): Stress creates a flight-or-fight response. This response increases breath rate, heart rate, metabolism, and the secretion of adrenaline. All of this is ideal when we're under a really serious threat. It powers us to safety or to fight for our lives. But most of the time we're not fighting or running for our lives, we're seated, or even lying in bed, anxious. This unused adrenaline puts us at an increased risk for anxiety, depression, insomnia, heart attacks, strokes, bowel disorders, infertility, and digestive diseases or issues. And these symptoms or diseases lead to excessive medication, via prescription and over-the-counter drugs. A majority of doctor visits are caused by stress. Can you believe that? The root cause for most visits to our doctors is because of stress.

Happily, we have an innate solution to the stress response: the relaxation response. It's a genetic set of changes that counteract the stress response. Meditation is *one big way* to bring about the relaxation response. Meditation can turn off genes that are inflamed by stress, especially useful for those with a genetic predisposition towards certain inflammatory diseases.

*"If you want to conquer the anxiety of life,
live in the moment, live in the breath."*

—AMIT RAY, Om Chanting and Meditation

*"If the problem can be solved why worry?
If the problem cannot be
solved worrying will do you no good."*

—SANTIDEVA

Meditation stops the mind from going over and over the same problems every day. Trust me on this one, I have a double worry line on my palm. But it's much fainter now. I've given up the worry habit, and meditation definitely helped with that. Meditation gave me the space and clarity to practice acceptance. Accepting something as it is, for me, allows for stress to recede. When new stressors arise, meditation helps activate the relaxation response, counteracting the stress, ridding the body of inflammation.

Inflammation is not complicated. It is the body's natural defense to a foreign invader such as bacteria, toxins, viruses, or stresses. The cycle of inflammation is perfect in how it protects the body from these bacterial and viral invaders. It works beautifully because protects your body against life threatening stressors. But most stress in today's world is not life threatening. You're not often going to be chased in the woods by a big bear. Most people treat the stress in their lives as if it's a big bear, claws out, ready to devour them. And it's the response to stress in our lives that shapes how much inflammation we absorb. Absorb the stresses of your life, skip sleep and exercise, and tell yourself meditation is for the annoying, crunchy granola girl in your spin class, not for you, and you'll keep that *chronic* inflammation level high. If we expose the body to injury by toxins and foods it was never designed to process—sugar, dairy, processed foods high in manufactured fats—*or by our response to daily stressors*, a condition called chronic inflammation occurs. Chronic inflammation is just as harmful as acute inflammation is beneficial. It's chronic inflammation that ages us and eventually kills us.

So, meditate. Help yourself to help your mind and your body.

Besides your daily meditation practice, another relatively easy way to assist in cooling down inflammation caused by anxiety is to reframe how you think about stress. Stress is inevitable; it is a part of life. So why not reconsider how you talk about the everyday, inevitable stressors in your life, because they will be there regardless. If you can put a positive spin on stress in your life, reframe it as a galvanizing force, you can change how your body reacts to it. The way we perceive stress, our perspective on life, and the way we react shows up on the cellular level.

In fact, reframing works as well in dealing with stress as it does with aging. It really is *the mind does matter*.

A 2002 study in the *Journal of Personality and Social Psychology* found that how we perceive aging affects how long we live. Those with more positive perceptions of their own aging lived an average of 7 years longer. You are what you think. Think yourself ageless. (Obviously, easier said than done, so act your way ageless too.)

Think about what you think about, especially when it comes to your daily stress load from work, family, relationships, commute, etc. How do you refer to work, your spouse or partner, homework, commute, bad weather, daily mishaps? Are you complaining? Harping on the negatives? Calling it a disaster? (That's my go-to. Everything from a missed flight to a boring yoga class is a horrible disaster. Wonder how that makes the rest of my day go? Hint: not well.) If you are constantly focusing on the negative you could be revving up your stress levels and aging yourself. Again, meditation works to counteract all this. It calms the mind, balances your perspective, and gives you clarity.

This idea of reframing our accepted concept of stress is something that researcher, teacher, and author Kelly McGonigal, of TED Talk fame, explores in her work. She suggests that instead of avoiding stress we reconfigure stress and what it means to us. How we perceive our lives creates the world we live in. Interestingly, our responses to stressors in life are often identical to how we respond to challenges. And, boy, how much do we love a good challenge? It's part of our cultural ethos. We view a challenge as something that makes us stronger, better, and, ultimately, happier. The idea is to "reframe the stress" into a challenge you have prepared for. The stress at work is like that triathlon you spent months training for (not that I've ever trained or competed in one of those, but I get the idea). You are equipped to rise to the occasion and meet the challenge.

A positive attitude is more effective in extending life than low blood pressure, low cholesterol, healthy weight, or regular exercise. This means if you do things to support a healthy, happy you, you'll have an easier time believing you're a vibrant, beautiful being, and this will in turn support an ageless you. It's a beautiful catch-22. A 2011 study in Biological Psychiatry found that aging success-fully is linked with a choice to live a happy, productive life, and to view the stress in life as character building, and as a tool to make effective change in your life. A transformation in your thinking can actually change how your genes express; they're the same genes, just different results. Like a big box of crayons, lots of colors but the choice of hue is up to you. When we allow past fears, stressors, and disappointments to rule our emotions and shape the way we experi-ence the present, we end up living and reliving the same emotional trauma without ever realizing it, creating new stress that our body absorbs, which is what makes us prematurely old.

CHAPTER 33

HOW TO MEDITATE

"Breathing in, I calm body and mind.
Breathing out, I smile. Dwelling in the present moment
I know this is the only moment."
—THICH NHAT HANH

Now, how do we get on that train to enlightenment?

In the beginning it's easiest if you create a meditation routine for yourself. After you've gotten hooked on the habit of meditating daily, then you can take your practice out for a spin and try it anywhere (except while operating heavy machinery or motor vehicles). But to start with, set a routine you can easily follow. Establish conditions for a meditation practice that will remain constant—the same time and the same quiet place. We have natural rhythms, and our minds and bodies respond positively to meditating at the same time every day. We also respond to the same visual and sensory cues. So, if you need to make your meditation practice a ritual, light a candle, fashion yourself a meditation cushion, listen to a guided meditation, and sit in the same place at the same time. Studies show, and neuroscientists have learned, that we form habits in a three-step "habit loop." It works like this: our brains prompt us to perform an act in response to a cue, like a meditation cushion or a lighted candle, we do the activity, we find it rewarding, which strengthens the loop, and then we become eager to do it all over again the next day. (I have an almost Pavlovian response at 2:00 p.m., when I usually meditate. I can't wait another minute to reboot and recharge. I am a creature of habit and routine. It helps me thrive.)

"Integrated meditation practice is like a healthy diet which is indispensable for maintaining your vitality and resistance to disease. Likewise, a balanced meditative practice in the course of a socially engaged way of life heightens your psychological immune system, so that you are less vulnerable to mental imbalances of all kinds."
—ALAN WALLACE

6 Steps To Get You Meditating

1. Choose a quiet space, your bedroom, your office with the door closed, the bathroom, your closet, a hallway no one uses. (I'm a big fan of my bed. Propped up by pillows, I sit comfortably.)

2. Find a comfortable seat. You want to feel comfortable and unrestricted. So if you're at the office, take your shoes off and your jacket. Get cozy in your space. Make yourself physically comfortable so that discomfort won't stop you from meditating.

3. Before you begin, set your timer for 12 minutes (or for longer if you want) so you won't worry about time.

4. Once you're seated comfortably, place your hands on your knees, palms up or down. (You can try the yoga way which is with palms up, and the thumb and forefinger touching. They say this completes an energetic circuit, and allows the energy to expand and rise in the body. But for me, it's not something I can often sustain for 12 minutes or more. So I keep my palms down.)

5. Close your eyes and begin with the breath. Allow the breath to flow in a natural rhythm. Breathe in and feel your belly expand, breath out and feel your belly contract. Breathe in, *get* present. Breathe out tension. Notice the gentle rhythm of

your breath as your attention becomes more and more set-
tled in the flow of the breath. If thoughts arise, let them rise
out of you without judgment, and then bring your attention
back to the breath. As the breath flows in and out, you might
want to breathe in peace and breathe out anxiety. (One meditation teacher I knew taught her students to see thoughts
that popped up as clouds, and watch the thought clouds float
away—good for avoiding judgment of the thoughts while you
meditate.)

6. If you need something to focus on other than your breath,
use a simple mantra. It can be a powerful way to enter the
stillness and to quiet your mind. You can say *Om* with each
exhale. Om is the most elemental sound for universal infinite
consciousness. Or, try *Ham sa*, which means "I am that." Or
you can find your own mantra, one that resonates for you.

And that's meditating in 6 easy steps.

If I'm doing a quick meditation while traveling I'll often use
a mantra. What is that? A mantra is a powerful sound or vibra-
tion that yogis have used to enter a meditative state. Here's Deepak
Chopra's definition: "The word mantra has two parts: *man*, which
is the root of the Sanskrit word for mind; and *tra*, which is the root
of the word instrument. A mantra is therefore an instrument of the
mind."

There are so many ways to meditate. I listen to a guided meditation on my phone with earbuds when I fly. I float away and tune
in to the silence of the mind while the soothing music plays. The
one I'm most keen on when I travel is Master Charles Cannon's
Synchronicity. Sheila, habitual meditator, turned me on to it, and
I find that the music is deeply soothing. It's an hour long, perfect
for most flights, or at home. I've also done the 21-day meditation
series with Oprah and Deepak as my guides. On our site we offer
several different approaches and audio guides to help you with your
meditation practice. Sometimes I find the easiest way to meditate is
by observing the breath—the inhale and exhale. Sometimes I'll use

a simple mantra, like *yum*, which is the *healing sound that resonates with the heart center*, but oftentimes I don't. I just let the breath, and the physical sensation of belly breathing, keep me in the meditative flow. In fact, you can use deep belly breathing anytime you're feeling anxious or bored. Try it next time you're at the DMV, waiting. Don't get frustrated with yourself or the meditation practice if it's not easy for you in the beginning, or even in the middle, because it is a practice. The more you practice and the longer you practice in your life, the greater the rewards and the more easeful it becomes. You didn't just wake up one morning and run a marathon, did you? Be patient and stick it out. I promise you it's worth it.

If you only learn one thing from this book, I hope it's how to meditate, because meditation is one of the very best things you can do for yourself and your world. When *you* meditate, we all benefit. Start your meditation practice today. There's no reason to wait for Monday!

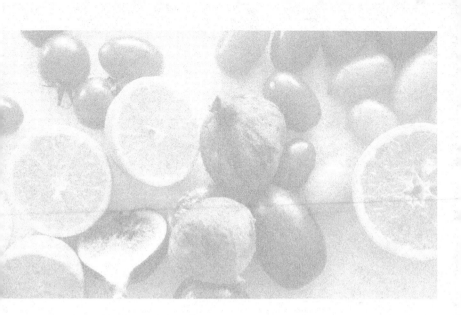

PART 4

Move

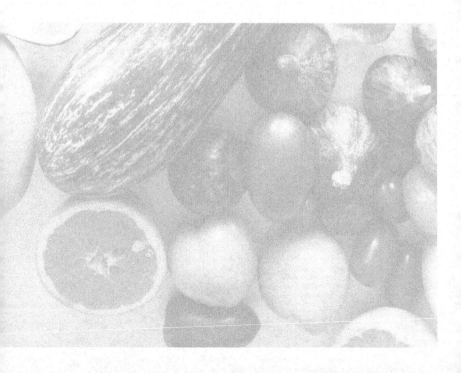

CHAPTER 34

WORK THAT BOOTY, AGELESS RULE #3

"Physical fitness is not only one of the most important keys to a healthy body, it is the basis of dynamic and creative intellectual activity."

—JOHN F. KENNEDY

The third Ageless Rule is physical exercise. Do some form of physical activity every day for those first 6 weeks. Move your body through space somehow, somewhere every day. That could mean a walk around the neighborhood, through the park, or around the mall. Go for a run, lift weights, practice yoga, take the stairs, dance around your room, do squats, try Pilates, Zumba, or a spin class, just do something—at least 30 minutes of physical exercise a day. It doesn't have to be a hardcore boot camp class, ironman competition, marathon or extreme Crossfit class, but you do need to move that booty. And give weights a try, adding free weights to your workout several times a week is a great way to build strength, tone muscles, and get fit.

Exercise every day for at least 30 minutes. After the first 6 weeks you can settle into a regular routine that works best for your lifestyle, take days off, have a long slow cardio day and short intense strength training session. Just make sure after the *6 Week Reset* you are exercising at least 4-5 days a week and varying both the activity and intensity. And savor the strength and grace of your own body. Moving your body brings happiness; there is great joy in movement. As Socrates put it, *"It is a shame for a man to grow old without seeing the beauty and strength of which his body is capable."*

There are four rules to the Ageless Diet, and there are four components to a healthy physical body: body leanness, joint flexibility, muscular strength and cardiovascular endurance. Regular, varied exercise contributes to all four of these healthy body goals.

Why is physical exercise so important? It boosts your mood and keeps the body looking and feeling ageless. Muscles become weak with lack of use. They look flabby and posture suffers—that's not a good look. Without regular physical activity the heart and lungs won't function efficiently. And the body's joints will be stiff and easily injured. Lack of exercise is as much a health risk as smoking. We were meant to move. We weren't built for sitting around all day. Getting fit reduces the risk of heart disease, cancer, high blood pressure, diabetes, and other diseases. Regular physical exercise is an absolute necessity if you want to be healthy. And if you want to be ageless, it's one of your top priorities. Plus, exercise is fun. It feels good.

The awesome benefits of exercise go beyond increasing flexibility and strength. Movement is so fundamental that when we don't move enough, all our body chemistry gets compromised. Exercise is essential for keeping your cellular energy at a higher level. And high cellular energy is absolutely necessary for health, longevity, *and agelessness.* We need to move and stretch those cells; it helps with the delivery of nutrients and the removal of toxins. Ever notice after a night out partying and drinking how bad you feel the next day? And then, when you finally go to work out, you can smell the old booze and greasy food oozing out of your skin, being sweat out of your body? I notice it every Sunday morning at yoga sculpt class. I can smell the type of liquor the guy next to me drank the night before. Usually, it's whiskey.

Moving and stretching cells addresses both deficiency and toxicity by facilitating the removal of toxins from our bodies. Exercise makes us happy. Cheapest and safest mood booster on the market! It's been proven to be much more effective than almost any anti-depressant out there, with the best side effects. Stronger core, weight loss, clarity of skin, improved cognitive function.

As you can imagine, exercise has a powerful effect on the brain. As with meditation, one very big benefit of exercise is promotion of new brain cell growth, which, obviously, is key in helping keep the brain young and in good repair. A 2012 study found that exercising as little as 30 minutes, several times a week, reduces the risk of dementia and the decline of cognitive skills by at least 60 percent. "These findings support physical-activity promotion campaigns by organizations such as the Alzheimer's Association and should encourage individuals to be physically active," study author Riu Liu said in a journal news release. "Following the current physical-activity recommendations from the American College of Sports Medicine (ACSM) will lift most individuals out of the low-fit category and may reduce their risk of dying with dementia," Liu added. What does the ACSM recommend? "'The scientific evidence we reviewed is indisputable,' said Carol Ewing Garber, Ph.D., FAHA, FACSM, chair of the writing committee (for the study on physical exercise). 'When it comes to exercise, the benefits far outweigh the risks. A program of regular exercise—beyond activities of daily living—is essential for most adults.' Adults should get at least 150 minutes of moderate-intensity exercise per week. Exercise recommendations can be met through 30-60 minutes of moderate-intensity exercise (five days per week) or 20-60 minutes of vigorous-intensity exercise (three days per week)." From the ACSM website. And, "it is no longer enough to consider whether an individual engages in adequate amounts of weekly exercise," said Garber, who is an associate professor of movement sciences at the Teachers College of Columbia University. "We also need to determine how much time a person spends in sedentary pursuits, like watching television or working on a computer. Health-and-fitness professionals must be concerned with these activities as well." Basically, exercise almost every day, vary the workouts you do, and avoid sitting for long periods of time. Consistency counts for the benefits both physically and mentally, and because no fitness program in the world works if you don't do it consistently.

And here are a few tips from the American Council on Exercise (ACE) for how to get fit:

1. **Strength training,** even 20 minutes a day, twice a week help tones the body. **Strength training** means using resistance to induce muscular contraction. This builds the strength, anaerobic endurance, and the size of skeletal muscles. Strength training improves your overall wellness, including increased bone, muscle, tendon and ligament strength and toughness, improved joint function, increased bone density, increased metabolism, and improved cardiac function. Strength training can include resistance bands, weight training, circuit training, and classes like yoga sculpt (yoga with weights), barre, and Crossfit. (I love doing a pyramid, which can go something like this: 100 squats, 90 Russian twist crunches, 80 lunges, 70 bridge lifts, and so on and so forth. The whole thing takes about 30 minutes, and leaves me stronger, energized, and sweaty.)

2. **Interval Training.** "In its most basic form, interval training might involve walking for two minutes, running for two, and alternating this pattern throughout the duration of a workout," says Cedric Bryant, PhD, FACSM, chief science officer for ACE. "It is an extremely time-efficient and productive way to exercise." Interval training could be when you vary your speeds and intensity during a short run. With interval training you can kickstart your metabolism within 20 minutes. (An easy way for me to interval train is to do *Tabatas* or *tabata training.* I do this when I don't have time for a long workout. Tabatas can be anything from burpees for 45 seconds on and 15 seconds rest to 3 minutes of high knees and 1 minute of jogging.)

3. **Cardio.** Increase your cardio/aerobic exercise. Cedric Bryant recommends accumulating 60 minutes or more a day of low to moderate intensity activity. Try walking, jogging, running, dancing, or climbing stairs. Get a device that helps you keep track of how much you move throughout the day. This encourages walking and moving more. (When it's cold outside

and I'm not going to make it to the gym, I turn on my favorite pop music and dance until I'm out of breath and sweating.
It's fun and easy.)

Physical exercise can ease depression, prevent age-related memory loss, and Parkinson-like symptoms, researchers reported at the
Society for Neuroscience meeting. Instead of doing all those cross-
word puzzles for brain health, go for a walk. Physical activity makes
you feel good, look great, and it helps keep your mind healthy and
vibrant.

"We definitely have more evidence for [showing the wide range
of brain benefits provided by] exercise," said Teresa Liu-Ambrose
of the University of British Columbia. She moderated a panel of
scientists presenting studies demonstrating all the benefits for the
brain that come from physical activity. As scientist Yong Tang of
Chongqing Medical University in Chongqing China, put it at the
Society for Neuroscience meeting: "Exercise, no matter how old
you are." It's daily rejuvenation, regardless of your age.

Exercise has been shown to "help reverse the Parkinson-like
slowing of movement that often come with age. The condition,
called bradykinesia, affects more than half of people who live to
be 85 or more and is responsible for many falls. The benefit may
come because exercise is raising levels of dopamine, a brain chemical that is important for movement, Jennifer Arnold of Louisiana
State University said," wrote Jon Hamilton for a piece on NPR. "A
pilot study of a dozen young adults in Australia found that exercise
relieves depression, said Robin Callister of the University of Newcastle. All of the participants, aged 15 to 25, had been diagnosed
with major depressive disorder. But after 12 weeks of exercise, 10 of
them were no longer categorized as depressed, Callister said. One
reason exercise provides mental benefits may be that it actually requires the brain to do a lot of work, Callister said. Even going on a
run means the brain is coordinating complex movements, she said.
And team sports or group exercises also activate parts of the brain
devoted to social interactions."

My favorite reason to exercise is that it feels good. I get a rush of endorphins and energy. Exercise is the one of the few things in life that gives you back more energy than you put in. It's a fact. If you feel low, tired, or depressed, physically and mentally, do a 30-minute workout and notice how much better you feel afterwards.

If you are moving your body, you're alive, because movement is life. And, in point of fact, if you aren't moving, you are dying.

Exercise, as with meditation, keeps those telomeres long. Exercise slows down telomere shortening. Physical activity protects your telomeres from the aging, inflammatory effects of stress. Proof of this from a 2010 study published in PLOS ONE about the effects of exercise on stress: "Vigorous physical activity appears to protect those experiencing high stress by buffering its relationship with telomere length. Chronic stress would be related to short telomere length in sedentary individuals, whereas in those who exercise, stress would not have measurable effects on telomere shortening."

Exercise delays the aging process. For this reason alone it's an Ageless Rule. Walking every day reduces the risk of an early death by at least 20 percent and the risk for cognitive decline.

"Exercising regularly is absolutely associated with lower blood sugars, on average, and it's also associated with brain health," says Paul Crane of the University of Washington.

But, let's not forget: it's impossible to exercise your way out of a bad diet. Just because you're working out regularly doesn't mean you can eat whatever you're addicted to. Foods like cupcakes, ice cream, cheeseburgers, and pizza are still bad news. Don't assume because you work out 30 minutes a day, you can gorge yourself because you "earned it." Exercise isn't an excuse to hit the drive-thru of your local favorite fast food place. You can work out every day and still be overweight because eating clean is 90 percent of how to feel and look good. But eating clean doesn't mean you can forgo workouts. Because we were meant to move; it's key to staying alive and ageless.

You may say: "Hey, I don't have that kind of time. And, even if I did, some days I just don't want to work out (or eat well or cook or meditate). It's not my top priority." Lose that way of thinking. It will make you sick, old, fat, and undesirable. Make physical exercise one of your top priorities. Show up for your health every day. No one else can take care of you like you can. Consider this, getting ageless and staying there requires taking care of the body and the mind, and that means physical exercise. It's a commitment, but you're worth it. I promise you will never regret 30 minutes of exercise. The little time and energy invested will pay you back in dividends; *you'll get more time added to your life and more energy back.* Keep it as low impact as you want, you don't have to be a warrior, you just need to move.

Think about this, we all have the potential to become fitness obsessed. On the days I don't feel like exercising, those are the days I'm happiest I did because I feel better. In fact, as someone who has spent years not exercising—ahem, college years—I know both sides of the workout coin. I've lived both ways, the one where a walk across the parking lot was my workout for the day, and the current lifestyle, exercising for about an hour every day. I feel 100 percent better exercising regularly. I used to be a depressive, no more. And, I have to confess, for me, it's easier to work out every day than try for three times a week. Once it's part of your routine, you're hooked.

So how do we, non-elite athletes, become fitness obsessed and tone our ageless figures? There are a few tricks you can employ to get you exercising daily. First, try working out at the same time every day, set up a routine you can follow. "Working out at the same time every day may help you improve more quickly, a study from the University of North Texas found, and other research has shown that people who exercise in the morning are more likely to stick with their workout than those who exercise later in the day," from an article by Amanda Macmillan. Second, working out first thing in the day saves you from losing yourself to distractions that seem to occur later in the day and cause you to miss your daily workout. Third, find something physical you love to do, a workout or an activity that helps you forget your worries and focus on the present moment. For me, that means group classes, like barre, yoga sculpt, or Pilates. And I love working with free weights in a group class. Join a gym (the local YMCAs in most cities are very affordable and typically have nicely-run gyms and class programs) or check out a yoga studio. Try something new if you're bored with your workout routine. Look for free community classes in your town. Find a group of friends and do a walk or run a few times a week. There are so many great ways to get a workout in, and there are so many options when it comes to physical exercise, it's easy to find one that suits your vibe.

If the word exercise or workout, bums you out, reframe your idea of working out, call it whatever word makes you feel good about doing it. Fourth, find an exercise that's near you, one that doesn't require a long schlep. Of course, this is from the person that used to take a 9:30 a.m. yoga class on 19th Street and 5th Avenue in Manhattan, when I lived in the bowels of Brooklyn, 35 minutes away by train. This brings me to my next point, if you find a class or a teacher or an activity that you really dig, you'll make the time and the effort to do it. The other bonus I got from traveling that far for yoga every day was the extra workout from the long walk to and from the subway. It was a wonderful way to start my day. And I got to see the people I liked practicing with me; we formed this community, and some of those people are now lifelong friends. And since in those days I worked late hours at a restaurant every night, I really needed the daily yoga class in the morning. Talk about an energy booster.

Because the *Reset* is 6 weeks, there's ample time to get hooked on fitness and to see and feel the positive results. So, just do it. I think you'll find it a big enough game changer that you'll keep it up. It takes about 6 weeks to develop a good exercise habit and to see and feel the positive results. Once you see these changes you won't want to go back to your old lifestyle and your old body. You'll come to crave the natural high that comes from a good workout.

In a 2006 study published in the *Journal of the American College of Cardiology* scientists showed a diet rich in whole foods, including healthy carbohydrates, fat, and plant-based proteins, **along with regular exercise** and not smoking, cools down inflammation. *Exercise cools down inflammation*. That's why it's an Ageless Rule. Because cooling down inflammation leads to agelessness just as chronic inflammation brings disease and premature aging.

We try and make it easy for you to get that workout in every day. On *AgelessDietLife.com* we have a variety of gentle to kickass workout videos to help keep you fit. You can do these almost anywhere, including hotel rooms. No reason not to exercise when traveling.

And lastly, and perhaps most importantly when it comes to working out, make sure you get enough sleep. If you don't, you won't feel like exercising.

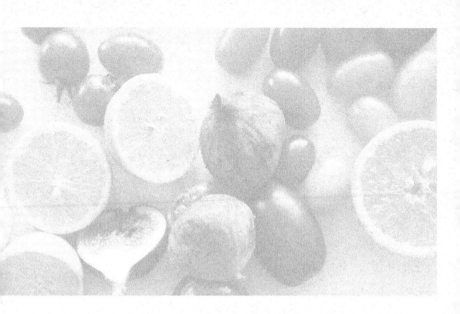

PART 5

Sleep

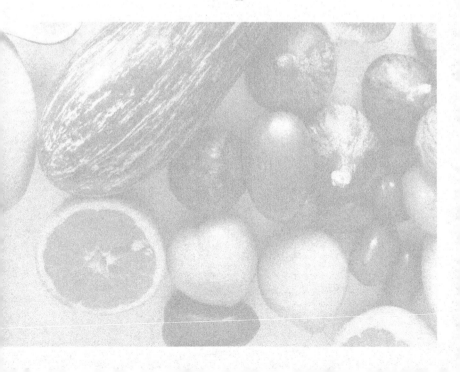

CHAPTER 35

AGELESS RULE #4— SLEEP!

"Sleep is the best meditation."
—DALAI LAMA

And now, the last Ageless Rule: a good night's sleep. Sleep is critical to feeling and looking ageless. Chronic lack of sleep can kill you. You need about 7-9 hours of sleep to rejuvenate yourself. I need about 8.5 hours, sometimes even 9. If you aren't getting 7-9 hours of sleep, time to change that. Adequate sleep is key to health, wellness, and happiness. It's time you honored your body's need for deep rest, and made it top of your list of priorities. (And if you're in the habit of not getting enough sleep, or not being able to sleep, there are things we can do to help you sleep.)

There are many very good reasons why sleep is an Ageless Rule.

A good night's sleep immeasurably improves life, and a life of little sleep will damage your body, brain, and work in ways you can't imagine. So privilege sleep above a workaholic lifestyle. You'll end up saving your employer and yourself money.

Why is lack of sleep bad for us? To start with, too little sleep can lead to weight gain. Chronic lack of sleep alters levels of the hormones that regulate satiety and hunger, leading to overeating and staying overweight. People who go through life with less sleep than they need tend to gain weight more easily, and the lack of sleep prematurely ages them. We tend to value work and the accompanying sleeplessness in our culture. We're proud workaholic insomniacs. I lived in New York, a place where people commonly boasted about needing less than 5 hours of sleep a night. It's why we're all so productive. But, maybe we're not. Chronic lack of sleep often makes us unproductive and uncreative, not to mention unhealthy. Sitting in the office for 13 hours a day does not make one productive, accomplishing tasks efficiently does.

Back in the day, when I was working at a restaurant till late, I was consistently sleep deprived. By noon, I'd be so tired I'd eat a big meal consisting of sugary low-fat muffins, sweetened yogurt, and fruit. And by 3:00 p.m., when I had to hop on the subway for work, I was exhausted. But even when I got home at a reasonable hour, around 11:00 p.m., I'd stay up till 2:00 or 3:00 a.m.. I told myself I didn't need sleep, and I was a happy insomniac. But I didn't have insomnia; I had bad habits. I didn't set myself up for success when it came to sleep. It wasn't until a year or so later, when I moved in with my first serious boyfriend that I started to sleep well. He believed sleep was important, and I saw he was happy and productive at work. I wanted that too. So following his lead, I started to sleep more. I slept 9 hours most nights. I learned from watching him that the more sleep he got, the better his day was, and the more he accomplished. And, by changing my habits, by really committing to a good night's sleep, my self-generated insomnia became a thing of the past. Most of us can change our sleep habits; we can become good sleepers.

You never adapt to sleep deprivation. You just get used to the negative effects of lack of sleep (the impaired judgment and reaction time, the bad mood, the weight gain, to name but a few), but your body never adapts to the chronic lack of sleep.

I'm not the only one to be poorly affected by lack of sleep. Sleep deprivation and overwork turned Scott into a gray-haired man in his early 20s. Long, lean, and lanky, Scott was on the swim team in high school, on track to become an Olympic swimmer. He rowed crew in college. He possesses the physique of a natural athlete, tall, broad-shouldered, and thin. But by his mid-20s he had a paunch, and he was fully gray. Premature gray is not a family attribute. Scott's expanding belly and gray hair came from extreme lack of sleep and the poor food choices sheer exhaustion leads to. Over a decade ago, in Aspen, Scott worked three jobs and slept with the lights on so he would wake 2 hours later for his third, morning, gig. He did this because he was chasing success, wanting to build his fortune, not realizing the sleep deprivation was aging him rapidly. And because of lack of sleep, all those years in college studying nutrition went out the window. It was all about eating whatever he could find whenever he had a spare moment to choke down food. His metabolism slowed, his belly swelled, and his hair went totally gray. He was a man in his mid-20s with a 45-year-old body. Now, at 40, Scott is lean again, strong, with glowing skin and a healthy metabolism. He gets enough sleep now, about 7 hours a night, and he's lost all inflammation. He has more stamina these days to accomplish what he wants, and the energy to exercise at least 4 days a week. He is also vastly more productive in his work than when he was just logging in hours at work. He's a young silver fox.

You can reverse the deleterious effects of poor diet, sleep deprivation, a sedentary life, all of which cause chronic inflammation. You can look younger in your 40s than you ever did in your 20s. I look better in my late 30s than I ever did in my 20s. So does Scott. So can you. It starts with a great diet and ends with a full night's sleep.

Sleep supports success; sleep doesn't snatch it away. The early bird catches the worm, but only if she goes to bed early too. If you're not an early riser naturally, honor that, and create a sleep routine that fits your natural rhythms. Sleep later in the morning, and build your work and life around that.

Sleep plays an important role in staying physically, mentally, and emotionally healthy. In fact, when I start to feel I'm getting a head cold, I try and get more sleep than usual. I'll go to bed early and fall asleep by 9:00 p.m., waking at 7:00 a.m., on the mend. When fighting a cold or the flu, scientists find that a good night's sleep can be one of the most effective cures.

What else does a good night's sleep do for you? Sleep is involved in healing and repairing your heart and blood vessels. Getting enough sleep is important for overall health because it's restorative, and it keeps you healthy and disease-free. It's as essential for your wellbeing as food and water.

Ongoing sleep deficiency is linked to an increased risk of heart disease, kidney disease, high blood pressure, diabetes, and stroke. Studies show that sleep deficiency alters activity in some parts of the brain, like those that control emotions, judgment, and reaction times. Sleep-deprived people tested on a driving simulator perform as badly as or worse than those who are intoxicated, and sleep deprivation is responsible for over 100,000 car accidents a year. You may have already discovered this on your own, and I certainly know it to be true for me. If I'm sleep deprived I'm not thinking properly. I'm more prone to be emotionally unstable, and my digestion is out of whack. Most humans react similarly when sleep deprived. It's been shown in studies that sleep deficiency increases difficulty in making decisions, solving problems, controlling emotions and behavior, and coping with change. It's also been linked to depression, suicide, and risk-taking behavior. Sleep is necessary for our nervous system to work properly.

As you may have noticed in yourself, too little sleep leaves us unable to concentrate the next day. It impairs memory and physical performance. Experts believe sleep gives neurons used while we are awake a chance to shut down and repair themselves. Sleep gives "the brain a chance to exercise important neuronal connections that might otherwise deteriorate from lack of activity. Deep sleep coincides with the release of growth hormone in children and young adults. Many of the body's cells also show increased production and reduced breakdown of proteins during deep sleep. Since proteins are the building blocks needed for cell growth and for repair of damage from factors like stress and ultraviolet rays, deep sleep may truly be 'beauty sleep.' Activity in parts of the brain that control emotions, decision-making processes, and social interactions is drastically reduced during deep sleep, suggesting that this type of sleep may help people maintain optimal emotional and social functioning while they are awake." (From the National Institute of Neurological Disorders and Stroke)

Sleep restores and rejuvenates. Without it we cannot function optimally.

The thing about losing sleep is that the more sleep you lose, the more you lose in life—opportunities, good health, strong relationships, happiness, etc. Most people these days are chronically sleep deprived, because it's become a vicious cycle. The less sleep you have, the less likely you are to privilege sleep, making it a priority, and then the less likely you are to get the sleep you need the following night.

Embrace your need for sleep because it feels so good. Support your sleep habit with the proper accoutrements since you spend a third of your lifetime doing it. Make your bed a place of comfort, invest in great pillows, good sheets, a firm, supportive mattress, get shades for your windows. When I slide into my bed at night, with the cool sheets and heavy down comforter in the quiet, dark room, it feels so good. I'm ready to fall asleep within 30 minutes of getting into bed. After I take my sleep support supplements, I read a chapter in a book, turn off the light, and slip into unconsciousness. I can't imagine not wanting to sleep. And when I wake after an 8 or 9-hour sleep, I feel like I've had the most luxurious experience. It's restorative in the way only sleep can be. It supports me throughout the day, powering me through work, life, and more. I'm less anxious and less susceptible to mood dips, depression, and anxiety. When I don't get enough sleep, tasks seem insurmountable, work is pointless, and life is drudgery. Of course, a quick half hour of exercise and an hour of meditation can boost my energy and mood on those days when I've not slept enough the night before. But nothing compares to sleep. It is one of our most basic biological needs. If we don't sleep we die. And before we die, we go mad. Why not indulge your need for sleep and rest your mind and body?

When you lose an hour of sleep your sense of wellbeing, productivity, health, *and* your ability to think decreases. If you want to be an ace at work, make sure your job honors your basic human need for sleep. Don't be a cowboy and operate on less than you require. It's simple math. We need sleep. It's fundamental to feeling and looking ageless. *And* it's instrumental in leading a successful, happy, productive life.

If you're feeling guilty for needing more sleep than your colleagues claim to require, comfort yourself with this fact: on average the best, most elite performers in the world sleep about 8 and a half hours a night. If the world-class performers need more sleep, shouldn't we need it too?

Sleep because you'll be better equipped to deal with stress.

Sleeplessness and stress have been linked to disturbances in the effects of leptin, the hormone that tells the brain that the body has had enough to eat. Sleeplessness and stress often go hand in hand. If you don't get enough sleep, you're more likely to react poorly to stress. Adequate sleep gives you the tools you need to react positively to daily stressors. It's not necessarily that stress causes you to eat more, but rather it causes you to gain weight by directly altering the activities of your cells.

"Sleep helps maintain a healthy balance of the hormones that make you feel hungry (ghrelin) or full (leptin). When you don't get enough sleep, your level of ghrelin goes up and your level of leptin goes down. This makes you feel hungrier than when you're well rested. Sleep also affects how your body reacts to insulin, the hormone that controls your blood glucose (sugar) level. Sleep deficiency results in a higher than normal blood sugar level, which may increase your risk for diabetes. Sleep also supports healthy growth and development. Deep sleep triggers the body to release the hormone that promotes normal growth in children and teens. This growth hormone also boosts muscle mass and helps repair cells and tissues in children, teens, and adults. Sleep also plays a role in puberty and fertility. Your immune system relies on sleep to stay healthy. This system defends your body against foreign or harmful substances. Ongoing sleep deficiency can change the way in which your immune system responds. For example, if you're sleep deficient, you may have trouble fighting common infections." (From National Institutes of Health)

Sleep deprivation also reduces your tolerance for pain. You feel more pain when you deprive yourself of sleep. And if you think pulling an all-nighter helps you seal that deal or pass that test, consider this, staying up all night actually reduces your capacity for studying and remembering new facts by 40 percent. Almost half of what you study, work on, and cram for is lost. Sleep deprivation is a major contributing factor in many preventable major disasters, including Chernobyl and Three Mile Island. You are helping save the world when you get the right amount of sleep.

Want to meet Mr. or Ms. Right? Get enough sleep. Sleep deprivation damages relationships. In a report titled *Sleep Matters* a link between insomnia and poor relationships, low energy levels and an inability to concentrate was discovered. The study demonstrated that people suffering serious sleep deprivation were four times as likely to have relationship and emotional problems, and three times as likely to feel depressed and suffer from a lack of concentration. If you're not getting sleep, it's hard to relate to people and attract the right kind of person into your life.

A senior researcher at Mental Health Foundation, in the United Kingdom, and lead author of the *Sleep Matters* study, Dr. Dan Robotham believes that poor sleep leads to a downward spiral, to mental health issues, which, in turn, trigger worse sleep. This is only one of many reasons supplements offering sleep and serotonin support are important. They help break the cycle, the downward spiral. And, the national epidemic is kind of a matter of national security. From the BBC News about the *Sleep Matters* study: "Professor Colin Espie, director of the Glasgow University Sleep Centre, said: 'We can no longer just ignore the impact of sleep problems in this country. They are affecting our health, our economy, and our everyday happiness.'" Think about that, lack of sleep affects our health, our finances (or lack thereof), and, of course, our happiness; it's been scientifically proven. And, if they think sleep deprivation is a serious issue in the United Kingdom, consider the United States. Americans and Japanese sleep the least. It's time for us to put our health, which includes our need for sleep, first. Because the truest thing I know is that if you don't have your health, you don't have much else.

We are largely responsible for our inability to sleep and for our chronic lack of sleep. But, good news, we can fix that. In a poll of people from around the world about their sleep habits, more than three quarters admitted to watching TV before bed, often in bed. This will definitely make it harder to fall asleep. In fact, many sleep experts feel that the excessive use of technology, our laptops, tablets, phones, televisions, is helping create a climate of sleeplessness. Most people struggle with sleep, and over 90 percent of Americans admit to using some kind of electronics within an hour before bedtime. These electronics mess with your production of melatonin, the major hormone secreted by the pineal gland that controls sleep and wake cycles. The artificial light reduces your levels of melatonin, leading to sleeplessness. And, if you're watching a stimulating program on TV, you get a hit of adrenaline from it. Do you really want to watch *Game of Thrones* or the nightly news or Jimmy Fallon before you fall asleep? Those shows are designed to stimulate, titillate, excite, and entertain you. Hardly what you need before you turn off the light and sleep. Keep TV and all other electronics out of your bedroom, and give up your late night TV watching, emailing, and reading on tablets. You will sleep much easier.

Sleep more because it gives you beautiful skin. Sleep deprivation, as with sugar, plays a major role in a premature aging and aged skin.

This may be totally obvious, but did you know lack of sleep is inflammatory and leads to faster aging—especially when it comes to your skin? A good night's sleep is instrumental to looking and feeling **ageless.** "In a first-of-its-kind clinical trial, physician-scientists at University Hospitals (UH) Case Medical Center found that sleep quality impacts skin function and aging. The recently completed study, commissioned by Estée Lauder, demonstrated that poor sleepers had increased signs of skin aging and slower recovery from a variety of environmental stressors, such as disruption of the skin barrier or ultraviolet (UV) radiation. Poor sleepers also felt less attractive; they had worse assessment of their own skin and facial appearance. 'Our study is the first to conclusively demonstrate that inadequate sleep is correlated with reduced skin health and accelerates skin aging. Sleep deprived women show signs of premature skin aging and a decrease in their skin's ability to recover after sun exposure,' said Dr. Elma Baron, MD, Director of the Skin Study Center at UH Case Medical Center and Associate Professor of Dermatology at Case Western Reserve University School of Medicine. 'Insufficient sleep has become a worldwide epidemic. While chronic sleep deprivation has been linked to medical problems such as obesity, diabetes, cancer and immune deficiency, its effects on skin function have previously been unknown.'"

Because skin functions as an important barrier from external stressors such as environmental toxins and sun-induced DNA damage, your skin is often the first line of defense in aging, and the first organ of the body to show aging. Hence, those fine lines and wrinkles, cellulite, and sunspots most of us despair over. Again from Dr. Baron's study: "The researchers found statistically significant differences between good and poor quality sleepers. Using the SCINEXA skin aging scoring system, poor quality sleepers showed increased signs of intrinsic skin aging including fine lines, uneven pigmentation and slackening of skin and reduced elasticity."

"Lack of sleep disrupts every physiologic function in the body," said a leading expert in sleep, Dr. Eve Van Cauter of the University of Chicago. "We have nothing in our biology that allows us to adapt to this behavior."

Sleeplessness, or sleep curtailment as the studies call it, is epidemic, and it's an accepted part of modern living, relatively harmless and necessary for maximum efficiency. How catastrophically wrong we are about that!

I know people who brag about how little they sleep. I used to! It's almost as if it's something they work at . . . becoming someone who operates on reduced sleep, like anything else, takes practice. The less you sleep over time, the more problematic it becomes for you to sleep. You're training yourself to be an insomniac.

And, what rewards do we reap from sleep curtailment? In a study published in MedScape, *The Impact of Sleep Deprivation on Hormones and Metabolism*, by Eve Van Cauter, PhD, *et al*, it was shown that sleeplessness is seriously detrimental to our health. "Sleeping and feeding are intricately related. Recent studies in humans have shown that the levels of hormones that regulate appetite are profoundly influenced by sleep duration. Sleep loss is associated with an increase in appetite that is excessive in relation to the caloric demands of extended wakefulness. Recent work also indicates that sleep loss may adversely affect glucose tolerance and involve an increased risk of type 2 diabetes. In young, healthy subjects who were studied after 6 days of sleep restriction (4 hours in bed) and after full sleep recovery, the levels of blood glucose after breakfast were higher in the state of sleep debt despite normal or even slightly elevated insulin responses."

You can reverse the negative effects from sleep deprivation. By simply sleeping longer and better, you can heal your body, your brain, and be closer to ageless. It's that simple, really.

> *"Sleep is the golden chain*
> *that ties health and our bodies together."*
> —THOMAS DEKKER

CHAPTER 36

HOW TO GET A GOOD NIGHT'S SLEEP

*"A good laugh and a long sleep
are the best cures in the doctor's book."*
—IRISH PROVERB

A good night's sleep may seem impossible, especially to anyone who has tried to sleep, tossing and turning all night, and can't. I know I've been there. I've had long nights with little sleep, and I broke the pattern. It's not hard to change your sleep habits. It just requires focus, patience, and time. In fact, there are a few simple things you can do to put you on the road to sleeping well. Even my insomnia-prone friends have benefitted from these Ageless Diet *sleep-more* tricks.

The best thing to do for better, longer sleep is develop a regular sleep routine, go to bed at the same time every night in dark room, with no electronics nearby. Make sure you go to bed early enough to get at least 7 hours. If your alarm is set for 5:00 a.m., adjust your bedtime accordingly. If you imbibe more than three alcoholic drinks a night, stop. Limit your drinking to more sleep-friendly levels (no more than two drinks). Move that phone you keep on your bedside table to an out of reach place, and watch TV in another room. Read a book before bed, and skip watching late night news or *The Tonight Show*. TV will rev you up and make falling asleep and staying there very tricky. The last thing any of us need before going to sleep is more stimulation. We live in an over-stimulated world, the TV is always on, our smart phones are always available, and we're online more hours than we're sleeping in our beds. So make your sleep life easier, simplify and keep all electronics, especially TV out of the bedroom. And for at least the first 6 weeks of the *Reset*, try the recommended supplements for targeted serotonin support.

Here are four simple things you can do for a good night's sleep:

1. **Go to bed at the same time every night. Create a sleep routine that works for your life.** (I take the supplements 30 minutes before bed, and thanks to a very simple sleep routine, I've trained myself to know it's time to fall asleep. When I draw the blinds, get into bed, and read a chapter from a book, by the time I switch the light, I'm ready to sleep.)

2. **Skip eating and drinking, especially alcohol, before bedtime. Eat at least two hours before bedtime.** Give yourself enough time to digest your food. And, don't go to bed hungry, it will keep you up. Drinking too much water will also keep you awake. No smoking. Nicotine and alcohol can act as stimulants in that they keep you up or, even more likely, disrupt sleep patterns. (I like beer or a glass of wine with dinner, several hours before bedtime, same with TV watching. I watch TV before bedtime, but not while I'm trying to fall asleep.) Alcohol may make you sleepy but that won't last, and you'll be up throughout the night. Don't forget for the first 7 days on the *Cleanse*, no more food after 6:00 p.m.—this should make sleep easier.

3. **Get rid of all electronics, including the TV, in your bedroom, this helps create an oasis for sleep.** Keep the drapes or blinds down and the room cool and dark. Make your bed comfortable.

"Life is too short to sleep on low-thread count sheets!"
—LEAH STUSSY

4. Try the Serotonin Support Supplements. Take sleep-targeted supplements for serotonin support a half hour before bedtime. (You can find out more about these supplements on AgelessDietLife.com.)

The great news is that by committing to this Diet, you are already enjoying a lifestyle that supports more easeful sleep. What you eat affects how you sleep, and thankfully you'll be eating clean, anti-inflammatory foods. You'll be meditating daily too, and that meditation during the day helps you sleep at night. The same is true with daily physical activity. Regular physical exercise promotes better sleep. A 30-minute walk or yoga class during the day can help you fall asleep faster and enjoy deeper sleep.

One more thing about a consistent meditation practice—I've found this true for me, especially if I do quick meditation before sleep—is that you benefit from deeper, more restful sleep and lucid dreams. You're also more alert when you wake in the morning.

As Rumi beautifully put it, *"Put your thoughts to sleep, do not let them cast a shadow over the moon of your heart. Let go of thinking."* Try a little meditation before bedtime. It's easy. You simply focus on your breath, doing abdominal breathing, in and out. Tune into your body. Continue being present in your body, breathing in and out while you sift through your day. With each event, review it and release it. With each action committed throughout the day, review and release. If you feel you've done something wrong or stupid, forgive yourself as you would your most favorite person in the world, don't go to bed holding a grudge, especially against yourself. After you've gone through your day, breathe in ease, breathe out tension. Take ten deep belly breaths and drift off to sleep.

And, definitely, for at least the first 6 weeks, take the supplements for targeted serotonin support. These supplements, including prolonged release melatonin, 3 mg (or more), L-theanine, 100 mg, GABA (gamma amino butyric acid), 100 mg, and passion flower extract, make falling asleep and staying there easier, without feeling groggy or tired in the morning.

"Melatonin plays a critical role in synchronizing the body's biological clock, and regulating its sleep-wake cycle. The rise-and-fall cycle of melatonin release is critical to our ability to sleep at night. A disruption in the body's ability to produce melatonin will lead to disordered sleep." From Michael Breus, PhD, Psychology. Melatonin can also be incredibly useful in dealing with jet lag successfully.

The other sleep supplements assist in quieting the mind. L-theanine is an amino acid that can significantly boost your REM cycles. Theanine literally shifts your brainwaves to a meditative state.

GABA is a neuro-inhibitory transmitter. The brain uses GABA to shut itself down. GABA, or gamma-aminobutyric acid, calms you and promotes relaxation. It also reduces anxiety. GABA is synthesized in the brain from another amino acid, glutamate, and functions as an inhibitory neurotransmitter—meaning that it blocks nerve impulses. In the body, GABA is concentrated in the hypothalamus region of the brain and is known to play a role in the overall functioning of the pituitary gland—which regulates growth hormone synthesis, sleep cycles, and body temperature. If you're feeling anxious, try a little GABA.

Passionflower (Passiflora incarnata) has been used for many years as a natural tranquilizer. Central American natives used it to sooth overactive nerves. It has been successful in helping with healthy sleep and muscle relaxation. It mellows you by boosting the brain's levels of GABA, which calms and lowers your brain activity.

I'm sure you've heard someone say: "I'll sleep when I'm dead." Yeah, sooner than he thinks. Don't be that guy. Sleep to live; sleep to thrive. Make this Ageless Rule a priority, and develop a sleep routine that works for you. It's time we started bragging about how much sleep we got, not how little.

CHAPTER 37

LIVE AGELESS
FOR EASEFUL LIVING

"What we hope ever to do with ease,
we must first learn to do with diligence."
—SAMUEL JOHNSON, *The Life Of Samuel Johnson*, Vol. 4

Living ageless is simple: swap out your current lifestyle for one that truly supports you. Nourish your body with real, whole foods you enjoy. Enhance your wholesome, healthy diet with a supplement program that helps to energize and revitalize you. Give yourself the gift of meditation. Exercise your body and your brain with daily physical activity. Sleep longer and better. All this may seem like work at first, but it's 100 percent easier than struggling through a day with the current bad habits that inflame, drain, and age you. Aren't you worth this effort? Don't you want to feel good or better or GREAT?

The more energy you put into your health and happiness the more you get back. And it's easier than ever; all the answers are in this book.

There are meal plans for you, recipes, shopping lists, and a supplement program. Check the site for regular updates. On Ageless-DietLife.com, we have workouts you can do anywhere, tips and guides on how to meditate and sleep well. And always, there will be new lists of foods, recipes, and meal plans to try. Most of the work is done for you. All you gotta do is commit to feeling better and looking great!

CHAPTER 38

AGELESS DIET ON THE ROAD

"It is better to travel well than to arrive."
—BUDDHA

Here are a few easy tips on traveling ageless. Travel and eating healthfully can be tricky. When I travel it's usually for work, and I don't always have immediate access to whole, organic foods. I also sometimes don't have the time to meditate or sleep more than a few hours. What do I do to stay ageless on the road? And how can you prevent yourself from going off the rails?

I love to travel. I'm not a once a week frequent flyer like some I know, but I'm typically en route to somewhere about two or three times a month. Pre-Ageless Diet, a trip to say Denver or Aspen to visit Scott meant all food bets were off . . . nachos, quesadillas, and big glasses of frosty Modelo beer from Su Casa, triple-frosted and layered cake from Main Street Bakery, doughnuts and other sugary pastries from the local patisseries, cheese burgers with hand-cut fries, rib-eye steaks with all the sides from Elway's, margaritas, martinis, and wine. Of course, my diet was already heavy in the high sugar but low-fat packaged foods, but when I traveled I'd use this as an excuse to indulge even more. It was easier than planning and schlepping good-for-me foods. Of course, with these relaxed standards came sleepless nights, wonky digestion, and a few recovery days once I returned to my New York apartment. Travel exhausted me. If I went abroad to India or France or even Mexico, jet lag was something I dreaded—it usually lasted at least 7 days.

Now that I live ageless I'm actually more sensitive and more prone to notice a bad reaction if I consume inflammatory foods like a ham, egg, and cheese croissant at the airport. It's one of those rules that can seem unfair, the healthier you become the more sensitive you are, like people who quit smoking and start getting every cold that comes their way. Most people think newfound sensitivity is bad. Who wants to be more sensitive to toxins in food and in the environment? I do because it keeps me healthy and happy. If I were unaware of my body's reaction to inflammatory foods and stressors, I'd get more inflamed and heavier without even noticing it, until one day I'd fall down sick with a serious disease. Heightened awareness is actually a good thing. Sensitivity to your surroundings keeps you alert, alive, and vital. So now, when I travel, I make the effort to stay on track, to live as ageless as I can. It's not as effortless in the short run as running to the airport, grabbing a coffee and a sandwich or buying a boxed meal in flight, but it's much, much easier in the long run. My travel goes more smoothly. I have more energy; I sleep better. I have no issues with digestion. I feel at least 80 percent better when I honor my body's need for good food, rest, and hydration.

A little preplanning on your behalf will keep you energized while you travel.

How do you travel smart while on the road, on a plane, in a hotel, or constantly on the run? Here are 7 simple tricks to *Traveling Ageless*:

1. **Pack Healthy Snacks.** Before you leave, pack a bag of nuts, or make your own blend (my favorite: currants, almonds, Brazil nuts, coconut flakes, and cacao nibs), a couple of organic apples and oranges. The fruit hydrates you, and hits that sweet tooth, plus they're full of fiber, which you need more of when you travel. I have a friend who always packs an avocado, with a little sea salt. He eats it on the plane. He cuts it with a plastic knife and eats it with a spoon. He loves the taste, and he gets good fat, fiber, and protein. If you love avocados, give it a try on your next flight. I also usually make a few sandwiches on

sprouted bread (if you don't have an allergy to gluten, try this too, and if you do, buy some organic corn tortillas or nori and make travel tacos). I make one with avocado, roasted tomatoes, pickles, and sprouts. I make another with hummus and tomato, and a third with almond butter. These sandwiches, tacos, or nori rolls are tasty. And when I get hungry I need to be prepared, because I make poor choices food-wise when the right food choices aren't around. You could prepare a chickpea salad with fresh vegetables and a mustard vinaigrette, or buy a half dozen of those travel sized nut and coconut butters. And, for a treat, bring a dark chocolate bar with at least 70 percent cocoa content. I like the ones with 88-90 percent cocoa. The nut butters are great for a quick burst of energy and protein. And the chocolate is good, because, well, it's chocolate.

2. **Hydrate.** Always bring a (BPA-free) water bottle and drink from it all day, and keep refilling it. Most airports now have filtered water near the water fountains designed for refilling water bottles. If you're driving, stop at a convenience station and refill your water bottle with water from their fountain drink stand. Stay hydrated. Drink more water than you think you need. The stress of travel often dehydrates us, and we need more water than usual, especially when in the air. Anytime the flight attendants come around with water, grab some. Staying hydrated helps you avoid travel lag, indigestion, and junk food cravings. Most cravings for junk food disappear if you drink a bottle of water. Aim for at least 90 ounces of water during travel days. More is better.

3. **Take Your Supplements.** You need the extra oomph that vitamin and mineral supplements provided. I flew to South Africa and back, a 36-hour trip each way, with minimal sleep—I don't sleep on planes—and I suffered little to no jet lag, in either direction. I land, go to sleep at the appropriate local time and wake in the morning refreshed and ready to go! I can tell you for sure that the supplements were key to an easeful

trip and a smooth transition home. They provide the edge you need when you're traveling. Consider them a necessary travel companion.

4. **No Junk Food. No Processed Foods.** More than ever it's essential to eat ageless when on the road. Avoid foods that drain your energy and deflate your mood. Stay away from juices, sodas, excessive alcohol, simple carbs, and high-glycemic foods. Skip the sugary snacks, cookies, chips, and pseudo-healthy foods like granola. And definitely avoid anything deep-fried. Skip sugar substitutes too. All those non-fat desserts and sweeteners are loaded with chemicals that your body can't easily metabolize. You don't need any of that junk! Anything partially hydrogenated (this includes non-dairy creamer, certain jarred peanut butters, margarine, and most packaged baked goods) will cause your energy to plummet, make your gut unhappy, and leave you craving more trash. Don't use travel as an excuse to cheat on yourself with junk food. You'll actually be punishing yourself. Remember, most of us overeat when we consume junk to feel satisfied. That usually adds up to extra 2,000 calories a day. As a pound of fat is about 3,500 calories, it means while on the road you gain weight. Stop the cycle of weight gain and inflammation before it begins. Stay away from fast foods, processed foods, packaged foods, and all junk food.

5. **Eat Clean. Stick with whole foods when eating out.** Make the staples of your diet these four food groups: whole grains, legumes, fruits, and vegetables. Opt for mostly vegetarian/vegan meals when away from home. Eat meals loaded with vegetables, which are much easier for our bodies to digest than meat. Buy salads with lean proteins, nuts/seeds, and grains. If you order a salad, make your own dressing with olive oil and lemon juice or vinegar. At restaurants, order steamed vegetables and doctor them yourself with a good fat like extra-virgin olive oil and fresh-squeezed lemon juice. You can even eat

clean at Mexican restaurants, try fish tacos or fajitas with corn tortillas, guacamole, black beans, rice, and salsa. That's one of my go-tos. At Japanese restaurants I order miso soup, seaweed salad, and salmon from the Pacific. At a steakhouse, I'll order a small grass-fed steak, baked potato, and steamed greens. Limit your consumption of anything containing alcohol to two glasses. If you're near a grocery store stock up on nuts, fruit, hummus, and fresh veggies. If I'm near a health food store, I'll buy their prepared salads and doctor them up with olive oil, tamari, and extra veggies. Anything you buy prepared, make sure read all labels. Try to stick with all organic produce. Use the condiments provided, like soy sauce, vinegar, and good olive oil to make the food taste better. Often when we're traveling, we don't always have access to food at regular intervals. PLAN AHEAD and keep your body happy and the metabolism revving with healthy snacks like a handful of almonds, a hard-boiled egg, one of my go-to sandwiches (avocado, pickles, and sprouts), fresh fruit, raw vegetables and hummus, and a little dark chocolate.

6. **Sleep.** As much as your trip will allow, sleep as long as you can. When I go to these integrative health conferences or film festivals I know for at least three days I'll be getting significantly less sleep than usual. So I make sure to slip out and meditate. It helps me feel and look refreshed. It works like a nap, and I can do it anywhere, on a sofa in the lobby of hotel. I keep taking the sleep supplements at night because they make a huge difference as well, helping me to sleep deeper. Energizing food and water can help replace lost sleep in the short-term.

7. **Move.** Pack workout clothes and running shoes. Your body, your mind, and your spirit will thank you if you take the time to walk around, do a little workout in your room, or hit the gym. You'll have more energy, which is exactly what you need on the road. (We have workout videos available online you

can do anywhere you have a little space and a wifi connection.)

The Recap: Stick with the **4 Ageless Rules**: skip dairy, wheat, and added sugar, sleep as much as you can, meditate, and exercise (even if it means walking up and down the stairs of your hotel). Pack as many healthy snacks, fresh fruits, nuts, nut butters, and simple sandwiches as you can, and drink more water than usual. Nuts are known as a longevity food. Eating 1.5 ounces of nuts per day reduces the risk of heart disease. It's also the perfect food on the go. Especially when on the road, eat 4-6 servings of vegetables a day. Take your supplements, and stick to a mostly vegan diet while traveling. Going mostly vegan is an easy way to eat clean. I do it when away from home, and you would be amazed at how easy it is and how good you feel. I still eat eggs and some lean grass-fed meat, but by eating 80-90 percent vegan I'm guaranteed healthier options. Take care of yourself so you can take care of business. And if you're traveling for pleasure, really take good care of yourself so you can enjoy every single minute of your trip.

CHAPTER 39

THE AGELESS DIET IN REVIEW

"Happiness depends upon ourselves."
—ARISTOTLE

Follow the 4 Ageless Rules and you will feel better. The side effects may include cellular regeneration, weight loss, increased energy, clearer skin, better moods, greater focus, renewed sex drive, and a toned body. If you can live with these side effects, try this *Reset* for 6 weeks. I promise you won't waste your time or your hard-earned money. There's no secret to being ageless, it's really, really simple:

The 4 Ageless Rules
1. Eat Clean.
2. Meditate.
3. Exercise.
4. Sleep.

A quick review of your first *6 Week Reset*:

Before you begin the first week of the *Reset*, the *7-Day Cleanse*, set yourself up for success by going grocery shopping for all the wonderful fresh foods you'll be lucky enough to eat these next 6 weeks, and do a little food prep to make cooking easier. Use the meal plan for the *7-Day Cleanse* to help get you in the groove. Get rid of all junk, sugar, and processed foods in your house. If it is in your house YOU WILL EAT IT. This will help you drop the inflammatory food and drink from your diet. Be open to new foods, especially if our recipes and meal plans include foods not usually in your diet, and incorporate your own ageless-approved favorites. Stock all the supplements you'll need for the next 6 weeks. You can make this step easier, if you want, by going on AgelessDietLife. com. If you'd prefer to source your own supplements, find ones you know to be good. Seek out the truth about what you're putting in your body.

Check out a gym or yoga studio with classes you'll enjoy. Figure out how to fit a daily workout into your schedule. Same for meditation; download a few guided meditations you think you'll enjoy.

And don't forget to have your trusty water bottle filled and nearby. Staying hydrated is a key component of the Ageless Diet, and drinking plenty of water will keep you energized and alive.

Week One: The *Cleanse*. Detoxify and cool down inflammation. Drop all inflammatory foods, including all processed and most prepared foods, dairy, ALL sugar, and wheat (and any grains with gluten). Add more fresh vegetables and fruits to your diet. Try the detox smoothies in the morning and afternoon, enjoy a real lunch, and a light supper in the evening, before 6:00 p.m.. No food consumed after 6:00 p.m.. Eat mostly plant-based. Give up all alcohol for this first week. And, drop coffee for the first 7 days. Instead, for a caffeine boost, try antioxidant-rich green tea. Set up a workout and meditation schedule that suits your current lifestyle. And commit to meditating 12 minutes and exercising at least 30 minutes every day. Order your supplements in advance and start taking them on Day 1 of the *Cleanse*. Observe how you feel. You should be able to tell how food affects you by the second week.

Week Two: *Reset*. Reset your diet permanently by continuing to eat clean, and eliminating all inflammatory agents you were consuming, especially dairy, wheat, and sugar. Stop eating an excessive amount of animal protein, continue with a diet that is 80 percent vegan, aim for eating vegan (no animal based foods) before 6:00 p.m.. Anything *inflammAGING* release it and let go. You're resetting your LIFE for GOOD. Eat clean, organic, anti-inflammatory whole foods, lots of fresh fruits and vegetables. In this second week, you can add coffee back into your morning routine, making sure to limit coffee drinking to before 2:00 p.m.. You can also, if you so desire, enjoy a glass of wine on occasion. Stick with wine and skip the beer for now. (After the fourth week, if you're not gluten intolerant, you can add back beer.) Keep up with a simple exercise regimen you can follow, one that fits in with your life. It may seem like a lot of change these first 2 weeks, with the supplements, cooking, shopping, food prep, working out, meditating, and sleep, but it works. You will feel better. In fact, feel yourself getting leaner, more energized, and happier.

Week Three: Lose Inflammation, Feel the Results. Congratulations! By the end of this week you will have completed 21 days on the Ageless Diet. Continue all your good work from Weeks 1 and 2, keep eating clean, and stay far away from all added sugars, dairy, and wheat, this should getting be easier as all the cravings subside. This is a perfect week to explore new and interesting recipes, restaurants, fitness classes, and meditations. Buy all your groceries fresh and take a few nights this week to really savor cooking for yourself. Step up your meditation practice by journaling a little after it, and notice what comes out of you and how you feel. Continue taking the supplements. After last week you should begin to feel and see results in your body and in your energy level. How are you feeling? Is your skin clearer? Are your eyes brighter? Join our monthly chat online. And, after this week, you can introduce a little dairy into your diet. Stick with goat milk, if you can, because it's easier to digest. And observe how your body is processing this food.

Week Four: Your Ageless Body. This week notice how you feel, how you look, whether you've lost weight or inflammation, are you sleeping better, are you thinking better, are you more able to handle daily stress, are the supplements giving you more energy, pay attention to YOU. And continue doing the things that support a happier, healthier you. Develop a breakfast routine that works for you. Which meal is your favorite? Start creating a repertoire of recipes you can rely on. Cook a few new ones this week. Have fun with your food. Food is medicine; it's also meant to taste good. Check out our site for another weekly meal plan, or wing it, you've got the shopping list, you know now what's ageless approved. Try out two new vegetables you have never eaten. Continue meditating, exercising, and getting 7-9 hours of sleep. And keep up with the supplements. On the first day of this week, Day 22, you can eat a little—not a lot—dairy, if you want. Be gentle with yourself, your body is clean, and you may react to dairy in ways you're not used to. If you want, though, and you have no allergic reaction, a modest amount of dairy is now allowed.

Week Five: Your Ageless Mind. On the first day of this week, it's time to reintroduce whole grains containing gluten. Stick with sprouted or long-ferment organic breads, or make your own bread! Have steel-cut oats for breakfast or another whole grain with gluten like rye or spelt or bulgur, and continue to skip the white and whole-wheat breads and any and all pastries. You want to observe how you feel when you eat gluten. Does it inflame you? Are you feeling worse or the same? If the same, you can continue with these whole grains and sprouted bread. You can even toast your gluten tolerance with an organic dark beer. Check out a restaurant in your town and enjoy a fun night out, celebrating new and different cuisines. If you want, follow our meal plan for this week, or make up your own, you know by now which foods you really love. Work out someplace new and keep up with the meditation practice. Continue with your supplement program and the sleep routine that works best for you.

Week Six: Ageless You. The next week of your life is all about fine-tuning the Ageless Diet so it fits into your life seamlessly from here on out. This is the final week of the *Reset*. You should know now how you feel when you eat dairy and whole grains containing gluten, and you should have a clear sense of which foods inflame you, and which foods make you feel energized and empowered. Because this is the last week of the *Reset*, really focus on these key things: *How are you feeling? How has your life improved? What would make your life even better? What do you want to manifest?* This week, when you wake, take 5 minutes and write a little stream of consciousness about who you are, how you feel, where you are, and what you want. Focus on feelings—how you want to feel. (And, if you want further insight, contact an intuitive counselor or consult a life coach. On our site we list a few of our very favorites.) You're open, you're eating foods that nourish and support you, your lifestyle is ageless, and you are vibrant. I strongly urge you to keep eating good food, sleeping, meditating, and exercising this week and in the following weeks, months, and years.

Your health and happiness is now it is up to you. Which new habits have improved the quality of your life? You *can* keep living this way, staying beautiful and ageless. The world needs more people like you, enhancing the Earth with your vitality and vibrancy.

It's that simple. Here's to you! Here's to living ageless and feeling better every year. Remember: You are Ageless.

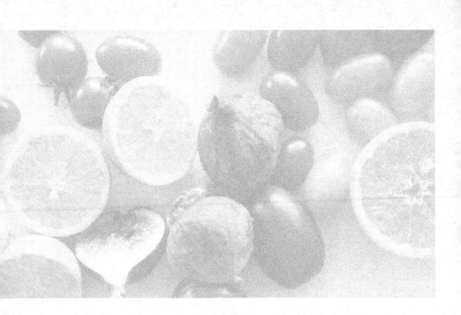

PART 6

Recipes

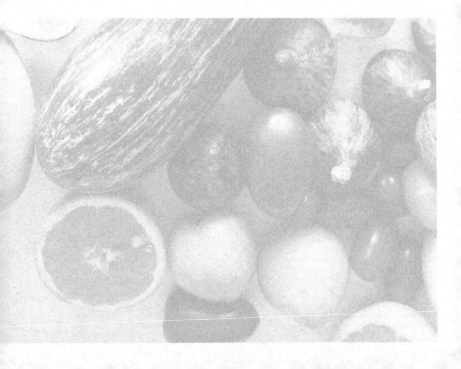

CHAPTER 40

MEAL PLANS:
A SIMPLE HOW-TO

"Did you ever stop to taste a carrot?
Not just eat it, but taste it? You can't taste the beauty
and energy of the earth in a Twinkie."

—ASTRID ALAUDA

Though I provide new meal plans regularly on AgelessDietLife. com, and have included the 8-day one here in the book, I thought I'd also give you some basic tips on how to plan your meals. I never thought I'd be one to plan meals for a week, or even a day. I love to eat guided by spontaneity and by what's available, fresh and local, at the Farmers Market. Now that I spend at least half my time in Colorado, cooking for more than just me, a year-round Farmers Market within walking distance no longer exists. There are great stores here for fresh food, organic, and varied, but for the meals I want to cook—ageless and flavorful, a little planning is required. Luckily meal planning is simple, and perfect for those of you with kids.

I plan my week's meals with my routine in mind. And I always make sure my staple of foods, those I eat every day, are on the list. My breakfast is cooking while I sip coffee, catch up on email, and peruse my pantry, fridge, and freezer, and ruminate on what I want to eat this week. Because I usually have the same thing every morning, I don't have to give breakfast much thought. I typically eat porridge of some kind, usually savory, and with steel-cut oats or quinoa. My very favorite breakfast is steel-cut oats cooked some-

times with quinoa, topped with blanched broccoli, celery, avocado, red bell pepper, cilantro, soy sauce, apple cider vinegar, toasted
sesame oil, and sriracha. All of which can be prepared and cooked
in less than 20 minutes. My lunches are simply assembled meals,
leftovers from the night(s) before, jazzed up with fresh greens or
a little dressing, an open-faced sandwich, two nori rolls, or a few
tacos with sautéed greens and black beans and avocado.

I also always need to have fixings for a kale smoothie, which I
enjoy in the afternoon. This means fresh pears or peaches, bananas,
oranges, parsley or mint, and kale. (Nowadays, I also add a tablespoon of maca powder, hemp seeds, bee pollen, and a big scoop of
my special metabolic boosting protein powder. Lily is gilded.) This
afternoon kale or detox smoothie routine also ensures I get to the
store for fresh veggies every few days. The kale-smoothie-motivated
shopping trips are great because I load up on other fresh fruits and
veggies that may be on sale, and have appetizing options for spur of
the moment salads.

Keep your routine in mind, and the foods you enjoy every day,
as you plan your meals for the week.

I draw up my meal plan on Mondays, because it's easier to shop
on a Monday than a Sunday, but if you have an office gig, by all
means, pick the days that work for you.

Before I do the meal plan I do these things:

- A quick inventory of **pantry, fridge, and freezer items** that
  I feel like (or that need) using. These usually include foods
  like eggs, edamame, frozen berries, Nama Shoyu soy sauce, fish
  sauce, peanut and almond butters, whole grains (quinoa, teff,
  oats, brown and black rice, millet, freekeh), spices, plus leftover ingredients or dishes from the previous week. (Do I have
  any lime peanut sauce left, or what about vegan pesto, or do I
  have tortillas and leftover guacamole in the fridge for a quick
  version of black bean tacos tonight?)

- The current list of recipes I've found that I want to test or foods
  I'm **inspired to cook.**

- A rough schedule for the upcoming week—are we going out to eat, any dinner parties we're throwing this week, is it a travel week, in which case I'll need to get mixed nuts, coconut, cacao nibs, extra apples and oranges, and make hummus for travel sandwiches, and which nights we're definitely eating in?

I review what I've gleaned from a pantry/freezer/fridge inventory. I scan the recipes I want to cook, and maybe do a little research on-line or check out a food magazine for inspiration (some weeks I'm craving certain foods like Thai basil beef, roasted chicken and root vegetables, a grass-fed beef burrito bowl, homemade sushi rolls, or a vegetable green curry with black rice), and then I make my list.

Here's what I end up with:

- A **list of dishes** and the days on which I plan to cook them, factoring in leftovers nights, which always occur, when I can use leftovers and a big bistro salad for a satisfying meal, and wild card dinners, nights when I'm too tired to stick to the plan or I'm craving an omelet or some other easy comfort food (my go-to meals: tacos, carne asada, a bistro salad with eggs, pota-to, legumes, broccoli, avocado, lettuce, and other veggies in a mouth-watering mustard vinaigrette, or squash noodle bowl with a lime peanut sauce).

- A list of **advance prep** steps that can or should be done the day be-fore (cleaning and chopping vegetables for crudités, for pad thai, new dishes, or for salads, soaking chickpeas for hummus or Mo-roccan vegetable stew, taking an item out of the freezer to thaw.)

- A **shopping list** of missing ingredients, with the days I'll be needing them so I know to coordinate the pick-up of these items with my regular kale-smoothie-fixings run to the store.

This gives me a **clear picture** of what we're eating for the week, what I need to do and when, and how much time I need each day (some meals take longer to cook than others). This also allows me opportunities to accommodate prep steps wherever they most readily fit in my schedule.

I love writing the meal plans for the Ageless Diet, because it's kind of what I already do for my household. They inspire me, get me excited about food and shopping, and give me a sense of the shape of things for the week ahead. So, if you find meal planning tricky, just go on the site and download that week's plan. My hope is that this takes the extra work off your already full plate and makes life easier.

(For more weekly meal plans, go to the site and subscribe to our weekly meal plan and recipe club.)

CHAPTER 41

EMBRACE COOKING

*"The only real stumbling block is fear of failure.
In cooking you've got to have a what-the-hell attitude."*

*"Cooking is one failure after another,
and that's how you finally learn."*

*"You don't have to cook fancy or complicated masterpieces—
just good food from fresh ingredients."*

—JULIA CHILD

Before we get to the Meal Plan section of this book and the two different shopping lists (one for the first 8 days and the second, a comprehensive list of everything you can eat on the Ageless Diet weeks 2-6 and beyond), I want to share some tips and thoughts on cooking. First of all, as I keep saying, embrace cooking. It's something we have to do if we want to eat good food.

Yes, there are days when I'm tired and don't want to cook. But I never regret soldiering on and making myself a quick meal. It's always worth the extra effort. And the easiest way to eat healthy is to get back in the kitchen and cook. Michael Pollan says what matters is, "not necessarily the nutrients good or bad of what we are consuming or staying away from, or even the calorie counts. But what predicts a healthy diet more than anything else is the fact that it was being cooked by a human being and not a corporation."

Cooking doesn't have to mean preparing elaborate meals. In fact, most of my recipes are quite simple and quick to make, with a few exceptions. But, I won't lie, there's no getting around the fact that if you want to eat well, unless you have a private chef, you must cook for yourself. Cooking can at times seem daunting, especially if it's new, but the need to eat necessitates some effort on our part.

If cooking seems daunting to you, remember this:

- Cooking is series of simple steps.

- Follow the steps and you'll end up with something delicious.

- The best food you'll ever make or eat comes from good quality ingredients, prepared simply. Spend more time locating fresh, seasonal produce, good grass-fed meat, or a pasture-raised chicken then rubbing it with a marinade.
- Relax when you cook, don't turn it into a chore.

- Fresh herbs make everything—everything—taste better. Use them in your smoothies, dressings, sauces, salads, etc.

- Improvise when you cook, substitute ingredients, and don't be a slave to a recipe.

- Guacamole always saves the day. When in doubt, make a big bowl of guac (and keep it super simple: avocado, lime, jalapeno, sea salt, and cilantro). You can eat it with any meal or as a snack. Guacamole on toasted whole grain bread or in a tortilla is a terrific lunch.

- After you broil or grill a steak (or any meat or fish for that matter), let it rest for at least 10 minutes.

- A squeeze of lemon, lime, or a splash of vinegar is a necessity to finishing almost every dish. It brightens all of them.

- I'm a big fan of lemon instead of vinegar in vinaigrettes. Try it. Having said that, I really dig the vinaigrette I make with sea salt, a splash of soy sauce, Dijon mustard, olive oil, and apple cider vinegar. The point is to mix it up, have fun with it. Make your own salad dressing. It's super easy. It's going to taste better, and it's much more affordable, with no danger of processed ingredients.

- Anything you cook is better than any prepared food you'll buy.

- Use the stems and stalks of herbs as well as the leaves. They are full of natural oils that impart amazing flavor.

- Clean and cut all your vegetables when you return from the market, storing them in a sealable container or bag. Doing this makes coming home and cooking that much easier and faster. Any task you can accomplish beforehand, on a free day, such as making dressings, hummus, bean dips, or chopping vegetables, that makes cooking a more easeful experience is worth it.

- Roast chicken is one of the easier dishes to make. Make this recipe part of your repertoire.

And consider cooking a form of entertainment. It's a pleasure, and aside from the health benefits of cooking our own food, it's one our favorite things to do. We've been doing it for millennia. It's a form of celebration and a way to create a sense of community. And, clearly we're fascinated by it. We watch so much cooking on TV. But it's much more fun and way more interesting to cook instead of watch. Give it a go!

CHAPTER 42

AGELESS DIET MEAL PLAN FOR THE FIRST 8 DAYS

*"Food, far more than sex, is the great leveler.
Just as every king, prophet, warrior,
and saint has a mother, so every Napoleon,
every Einstein, every Jesus has to eat."*
—BETTY FUSSELL, Author of *My Kitchen Wars*

This meal plan for your first 8 days is a guide, as is the shopping list. If you discover a dish you really love, like the Bistro Salad, or find you could eat hummus (check the site for a great hummus recipe) and avocado every day—make a tortilla or nori wrap with that and add fresh greens. Let what you love dictate what you eat. And, if like me, you could eat the same breakfast every day—savory porridge with fresh vegetables—then do that. Though, for the first 8 days, I think you'll find the smoothies quite filling, and will probably want a lighter breakfast (a handful of nuts or a plate of fresh fruit). Basically do what works best for you and your tastes within the parameters of the *Cleanse* and *Reset*. And, if you seek variety in your diet, I think you'll be happy with this meal plan. Recipes to most of the suggested dishes are below this 8-Day Meal Plan. (You can find the rest on the site.) Please note: Most recipes for this meal plan will serve 2-4. If you doing the *Cleanse/Reset* solo, feel free to adapt each recipe to your serving requirements. You can make more labor intensive recipes (soups, dressing, meat marinades) in advance and enjoy those dishes for lunch and dinner 2 days in a row. Bottom line: make this your meal plan and choose your favorites from the options provided. And, stick to the rules: no sugar, no dairy, and no wheat.

Quick bullet points before we hit the 8-day Meal Plan:

1. Prep before you start the Ageless Diet, go shopping, make some recipes ahead, chop vegetables for the week, and set yourself up for success. Roast a chicken on Sunday or pick an organic one up at the store mid-week for easy, quick meals.

2. Be flexible. If you have leftovers from dinner, make lunch with them, adding a quick and easy green salad. After that first week, if you go out for dinner, order smart, avoid the Big 3: sugar, dairy, wheat.

3. Have fun, get creative, if you want, or stick to the meal plan. If there's a grain, seed, nut, protein, or vegetable you love, add that. If there are foods you don't like, substitute. The point is to prepare food that tastes good to you.

4. Start every morning with a glass of filtered water and fresh juice from half a lemon. This refreshes you and helps cleanse the liver.

Comprehensive Shopping List for Week 1

(Some of these items will last through the weeks of the *Reset*. Because, we're also stocking your pantry. And, of course, this list can be amended or augmented to suit your tastes, family, and serving sizes.)

4 cans of organic black beans

1 can of cannellini beans for quick salads

1 pound of red lentils

2 cans of chickpeas

Dijon or whole grain mustard

Soy sauce or tamari

Unfiltered apple cider vinegar

Rice wine vinegar

Hot sauce: sriracha, chile paste, cholula

Worcestershire sauce (for steak salad marinade)

Fish sauce or oyster sauce

Extra-virgin olive oil (EVOO)

Safflower, sunflower, or peanut oil

Toasted sesame oil

Sea salt

Cumin

Smoked paprika

Cinnamon

Ground coriander

Ground cayenne pepper

Dried herbs (oregano, thyme, marjoram)

4 bags of frozen berries (blackberry, strawberry, blueberry, and raspberry) for smoothies

Raw nuts & seeds (almonds, cashews, walnuts, brazil nuts, pine nuts, pumpkin seeds, etc.)

Chia seeds

Hempseeds

Flaxseeds

Maca powder (for superfood green smoothie, optional)

Bee Pollen (for superfood green smoothie, optional)

Cacao nibs (for chia seed pudding)

Almond milk (UNSWEETENED, plain) or another unsweetened plant or nut-based milk (you can easily make your own almond milk, recipe in this book)

Plant-based protein (unsweetened, organic, plain)—optional, if you want to add to your smoothies for extra heft (for smoothies as meal replacement)—can substitute hemp seeds for powder

Almond butter or peanut butter (unsweetened, organic)

Tahini (sesame seed paste)

Nutritional Yeast

Quinoa

(*optional*) Millet or other gluten-free whole grains (for grain bowls)

(*optional*) Brown or Black Rice (for grain bowls)

Nori (sheets of dried, toasted seaweed)

Corn tortillas (sprouted, organic preferably)

1 medium-sized butternut squash

Arugula and/or Frisée

Broccoli

Cabbage (for quick salads, slaws, and you can use the cabbage leaves for tacos)

Zucchini (for salads and quinoa bowl with summer produce)

Cucumbers (3-4)

Kale (3 bunches)

Spinach, watercress, or chard

Fresh herbs (oregano, rosemary, thyme, your favorites)

Basil

Mint

Parsley (2 bunches)

Cilantro (2 bunches)

Lettuce (romaine, red leaf, and/or butter)

Sprouts (mung bean, sunflower, kaiware, alfalfa, broccoli, spicy radish)

Microgreens

2 fat bulbs of garlic

Onions (yellow, red, and white)

Scallions

Red and yellow bell peppers (2-3)

Hot peppers (jalapeño, poblano, anaheim, Serrano chiles)

1 bunch or 1 pound of carrots (for salads, rolls, and snacks with hummus or baba ghanoush)

2 stalks of celery

Mushrooms (for sautéing, in bistro salad and in omelet)

Brussels sprouts

Oranges (at least 6, if I make a kale smoothie for 2 people, I use 2 oranges daily)

Apples (for snacks)

Pears, Peaches, Nectarines

Bananas (for snacks and smoothies)

Avocados (at least 3)

Grape/cherry tomatoes (for salads, if you want)

6 tomatoes or bigger ones for burritos, black bean recipes, tomato & red lentil soup

Lemons (at least 6)

Limes (at least 4)

1 dozen pasture-raised, organic eggs

1 organic, pasture-raised whole chicken (to roast) or a store-bought organic roast chicken—a roasted chicken is handy to have around for quick lunches and dinners (with a whole grain and steamed or sautéed greens, shredded chicken with a citrus dressing is terrific)

(*optional*) 2 cans of wild, pole-caught Alaskan salmon or trout salmon (packed in oil) for quick salads or sandwiches (mix the salmon or tuna with olive oil, mustard, vinegar, salt, pepper, serve in salad wraps made from cabbage leaves)

Smoked salmon or trout (for nori rolls with salmon or trout)

Naturally fermented pickles, sauerkraut, kimchi, or any other pickled vegetable you love

Meal Plan Option 1
Endless variations of these
4 dishes for breakfast, lunch or dinner

• Egg dishes (poached, fried or omelets) with fresh, steamed, or sautéed greens

• Savory Porridge/Grain Bowls

• Big Bistro Salads

• Tacos & Nori Rolls

Meal Plan Option 2
The 8-Day Meal Plan

DAY 1
Breakfast Detox AM Smoothie with fresh fruit and ¼ cup raw nuts

Lunch 2-3 Raw Vegan Nori Rolls with tahini & nutritional yeast

Mid-afternoon snack Detox PM Smoothie

Dinner Roast chicken with quinoa tabbouleh
Suggestion: When making quinoa tabbouleh save some for lunch and cook an extra ½ cup of quinoa for breakfast

DAY 2
Breakfast Detox AM Smoothie and fresh fruit drizzled with almond butter and cinnamon (warm 2 tablespoons of almond butter in a pan before drizzling)

Lunch Chickpea salad with quinoa tabbouleh

Mid-afternoon snack Detox PM Smoothie

Dinner Mushroom & Fresh Herb Omelet with a green salad

DAY 3
Breakfast Detox AM Smoothie

Lunch Green salad with cannellini beans. (Chopped arugula or spinach with 1 can drained, rinsed cannellini beans, ½ avocado chopped, minced red onion, capers, olive oil, fresh lemon juice, finely chopped fresh flat-leaf or Italian parsley. Toss this salad, and spoon this mixture onto butter or romaine lettuce or green cabbage if you want to make lettuce/cabbage wraps. Season to taste with salt and pepper.)

Mid-afternoon snack Detox PM Smoothie

Dinner Ginger soy citrus salmon (if cooking salmon, marinate this for at least 3 hours, and reserve some for tomorrow's lunch) with broccoli and edamame salad

DAY 4
Breakfast Detox AM Smoothie

Lunch 2-3 Nori Rolls with leftover salmon or smoked salmon/ trout and sesame dipping sauce

Mid-afternoon snack Detox PM Smoothie

Dinner Fresh Tomato, Red Lentil Soup

DAY 5
Breakfast Detox AM Smoothie

Lunch Tomato lentil soup (leftovers from dinner) with a few carrot sticks for crunch

Mid-afternoon snack Detox PM Smoothie

Dinner Butternut Squash Chickpea Salad with Arugula

DAY 6
Breakfast Detox AM Smoothie with a handful of raw nuts

Lunch 2 Tacos—you can make a taco out of almost anything. Use organic corn tortillas (they are available almost everywhere these days), fill it with fresh greens, sprouts, leftover black beans, salmon or shredded roast chicken, avocado, sautéed kale, or anything else you enjoy.

Mid-afternoon snack Detox PM Smoothie

Dinner Chinese Chicken Salad

DAY 7

Breakfast Detox AM Smoothie

Lunch 2-3 Raw Vegan Nori Rolls (can be made in the morning and kept in an airtight container until lunchtime)

Mid-afternoon snack Detox PM Smoothie

Dinner Bistro Salad

DAY 8:
(you can have coffee and wine if you want now, and eat food after 6:00 p.m.)

Breakfast Superfood Green Smoothie and Chia Pudding

Lunch Salmon Salad with mustard vinaigrette (1 can of wild-caught salmon, chopped celery, red onion, mustard vinaigrette, served over arugula or spinach with ½ avocado, and fresh herbs—parsley, basil, mint, or dill work best)

Mid-afternoon snack Kale Smoothie

Dinner Black Beans—instead of rice, serve the beans with a green salad. (This is a quick 15-minute dish to make, and if you find yourself pressed for time later or earlier in the week, make this your go-to dinner dish. I could almost eat it every night.)

Note: For all recipes listed on the meal plan but not provided in the next chapter, please go to AgelessDietLife.com. All recipes for the meal plans are on the site, free and available to all.

CHAPTER 43

AGELESS DIET RECIPES

"I hate the notion of a secret recipe.
Recipes are by nature derivative and meant to
be shared—that is how they improve,
are changed, how new ideas are formed. To stop a recipe
in its tracks, to label it 'secret' just seems mean."

—MOLLY WIZENBERG

Here are a handful recipes, tested and verified healthy, delicious, and ageless, to prepare while on the *6 Week Reset*. I cook most of these recipes and the others, found on the site, sometimes daily and at the very least, a couple of times a month. At least in the beginning, especially the first 3 weeks, it's easier, cheaper, and better for your overall wellness, if you cook and prepare your own foods. It gets you in touch with what you eat, how you eat, and the food system you're a part of. Are you supporting a food system that supports you and the planet or are you subsidizing unhealthy habits and industrialized farming? The easiest way to change your diet and control what you eat is to cook your own food. It puts you in direct contact with the food you eat. Vote with your pocketbook and support organic, local farms, and buy local and organic.

SMOOTHIES

DETOX SMOOTHIES (AM & PM)

All the ingredients in these smoothies are power-packed with anti-inflammatory nutrients. They taste good and supercharge you. Start your morning with this Detox AM Smoothie, it's filling enough that you can drink this and run out the door.

Morning Detox Smoothie

(serves 2)

1/2 cucumber

2 cups frozen berries (mix of raspberries, blueberries, strawberries, and blackberries)

5 leaves of kale with stems, cleaned, chopped, or 1 cup packed spinach

1 scoop of Ageless *Cleanse* + Detox protein powder (or a plant-based protein powder—pea, rice, or hemp—of your choice)

½ cup unsweetened (homemade) almond milk (or a plant-based milk of your choice)

1 banana

1 lemon, peeled and chopped

(Optional) I tablespoon hempseeds or ground flaxseeds

1. Chop the vegetables and fruits into bite-sized chunks. Allow the berries to defrost enough so that they blend easily.

2. Blend the banana, berries, lemon and protein powder with the almond milk and just enough water to cover. If using, add hempseeds or flaxseeds.

3. Add the cucumber, and kale. Blend until smooth. You shouldn't need ice because the berries are still slightly frozen.

4. Pour into glasses or an opaque container and enjoy!

Afternoon Detox Smoothie
(serves 2)

1 celery stick, chopped

1/2 cucumber, chopped

1 peach or pear or nectarine

1/2 cup fresh or frozen blueberries

1 orange, peeled

3 big leaves of kale with the stems, chopped

1 cup watercress, chard, or spinach, chopped

1/4 cup mint or parsley

1 tablespoon hempseeds or ground flaxseeds

1. Chop the celery, cucumber, kale, and peach/pear/nectarine into bite-sized pieces. Divide the orange into individual segments.

2. In a blender, blend the berries, peach/pear/nectarine, and orange with enough water to cover it.

3. Add the kale, watercress/spinach/chard, cucumber, celery, and mint or parsley to the blender. Add hempseeds. Blend until smooth.

4. Add enough ice, about 4-5 cubes (1 cup) to make the smoothie cold.

5. Serve in a tall glass or make in the morning and keep in an opaque container, saving it for your mid-afternoon snack. Enjoy!

Note: watercress has a very peppery taste, if you prefer a milder green, stick with spinach or chard

Kale Smoothie

(serves 2)

A simple recipe of organic kale, pear, orange and mint. Put in your blender, blend until smooth, drink. You'll feel better immediately!

1 Bunch of organic kale (Red, Green, Tuscan, or Lacinato)

1 Pear

2 oranges

5-7 sprigs of mint (or parsley)

8-10 oz. of water

Ice

1. Peel oranges, chop into segments, add to blender. Core the pear and add to blender. Add water to cover (approximately 10 oz. or 2/3 cup water). Blend until smooth.

2. Add mint. Blend.

3. Chop kale, slowly add to blender, blending the whole time, add water as needed. Blend until smooth (depending on how powerful your blender is you may need to blend longer and add more water). Add ice (about ½ a glass). Blend for 15 seconds.

4. Pour into 2 glasses. Serves 2 people with a little extra.

*Note: this is a great recipe to make your own, add what you love, play with it, make it to your taste. Sometimes I add 2 peaches, 1 orange, and a bunch of parsley. And other times I use half chard, half kale, add a lemon with the orange, and pear. If blood oranges are in season those are great to use. My mother uses Texas Pete's hot sauce. The point is to make it your own.

Superfood Green Smoothie
(serves 2)

2 cups chopped kale

1 banana, peeled, chopped

2 cara cara or blood oranges, peeled, cut into segments

1/2 cup unsweetened almond milk (or a nut milk of your choice, brazil nut milk is a good option)

2 tablespoons hemp seeds

1 tablespoon bee pollen

2 teaspoons maca powder

Filtered water (about 1 cup)

Ice (about 1 cup)

1. Add all the ingredients to the blender, with barely enough water to cover. (You want a little, creamy smoothie, not a watery, thin one.)

2. Blend until smooth.

3. Add the almond milk and ice. Blend for another 20 seconds or so.

4. Serve in 2 big glasses.

Homemade Almond Milk

(yields 2 ½ cups)

1/2 cup whole raw almonds

1/2 teaspoon vanilla extract

Pinch ground cinnamon

Pinch coarse salt

1. Place almonds in a small bowl and cover with 2 inches of water. Let soak overnight in refrigerator.

2. Drain almonds and remove skins with a paring knife. Discard skins. Transfer to a blender and add 2 cups water, vanilla, cinnamon, and salt. Blend on high speed for 1 minute.

* *Note*: This will keep refrigerated for about 5 days.

BREAKFAST

Chia Seed Pudding

Chia seed pudding is super simple to make; there's no cooking required. Mix one part chia seeds with two parts liquid (almond milk is probably the easiest choice), stir, and wait. Over the course of 15 to 30 minutes, the chia seeds will gelatinize and the pudding will thicken up nicely. You can use your favorite plant or nut-based milk, just make sure it's organic and unsweetened. And, you can add whatever fruit and nut combination you like to this pudding. It's rather bland, so I like to jazz it up with raspberries, nuts, cacao nibs, goji berries, raisins, pomegranate seeds, cinnamon, a few tablespoons of hempseeds, and anything else I can think of for extra flavor. A breakfast made with chia seeds, fresh fruits, nuts, and cacao nibs is an antioxidant powerhouse of a breakfast. Chia seeds are high in omega-3s, and they are an excellent source of calcium, phosphorus, magnesium, potassium, iron, zinc, and copper. They have a high protein composition (19-23%) too, making them a kind of perfect food.

Basic Chia Seed Pudding Recipe
(yields 3-4 servings)

3/4 cup chia seeds

2 cups unsweetened, organic almond milk

Sea salt

(for 1 serving)

2 tablespoons chia seeds

1/2 cup almond milk (or any other plant-based milk you like)

Sea salt (about 1/4 teaspoon)

Simply mix the ingredients together, and let the mixture rest for 10 minutes. Stir again and after 5 minutes serve.

Raspberry Cacao Chia Pudding Recipe
(yields 3-4 servings)

3/4 cup chia seeds

2 cups unsweetened, organic almond milk

1 teaspoon sea salt

2/3 cup cacao nibs

1 cup raw walnuts

(optional) 3 tablespoons hempseeds

2 cups fresh raspberries

In a bowl mix the chia seeds, sea salt, and almond milk together, and let the mixture rest for about 10 minutes. Stir again until the consistency is smooth and pudding like, let rest another 5 minutes. After about 15 minutes total, serve in bowls. Top each chia pudding bowl with fresh raspberries, walnuts, hempseeds, and cacao nibs. Enjoy!

Savory Porridge

(serves 2)

For the first 28 days on the *Reset,* use only quinoa or another gluten-free grain, skip the steel-cut oats, unless you have access to gluten-free oats.

2 1/2 cups of water

1/2 cup organic steel-cut oats

1/2 cup organic quinoa

1 big stalk broccoli (use the stem and the crown in this dish), blanched, chopped

1/2 bunch cilantro, chopped

4 teaspoons of toasted sesame oil (or olive oil)

2 teaspoons of soy sauce, plus more to taste

1/2 teaspoon sea salt

Big splash of apple cider vinegar (about a tablespoon for each bowl), more to taste

Sriracha to taste

Note: Feel free to add any other fresh vegetables you love: red and yellow bell peppers, spinach, kale, edamame, avocado, carrots, celery, kohlrabi, bok choy . . . the options are endless. A combo of red bell pepper, celery, cucumber, avocado, cilantro, and broccoli is divine. Do try to use all organic ingredients if possible and available.

1. Put 2 1/2 cups of water with a 1/2 teaspoon of sea salt in a pot, bring to a simmer, add the oats and quinoa, or just 1 cup of quinoa, reduce heat to a very low flame. Cook for about 20 minutes. Remove the pot from the heat once done.

2. While the porridge cooks, blanch the broccoli. Allow to cool and then chop the stalk and crown into bite-sized pieces. Chop the cilantro.

3. Spoon the porridge into two bowls, drizzle each with about 2 teaspoons of sesame oil and soy sauce—add a little more of both, if you want the dish to be a little richer tasting. Top with the broccoli and cilantro (and other veggies, if you're adding more). Squeeze fresh lime juice on top and Sriracha if you want it spicy.

ENTRÉES

Quinoa Veggie Bowl
(serves 4)

2 tablespoons olive oil

2 tablespoons sherry or red wine vinegar

2 tablespoons Dijon mustard, or to taste

Fresh lime juice, about 1/2 a lime

1 teaspoon salt

1 teaspoon pepper

1 large shallot or small red onion, chopped

1 teaspoon minced garlic

3 cups cooked quinoa

1 large red bell pepper, chopped

1 cup zucchini (roasted or raw), chopped

2 cups corn kernels, preferably fresh

1 pint cherry or grape tomatoes, halved

1 cup fresh basil, chopped

1/2 cup fresh mint, chopped

1. Whisk together the oil, vinegar, mustard, salt, and pepper with 2 tablespoons water in a large bowl. Add the red onion and garlic, whisk again, and taste. Add more mustard, salt, and pepper if you like.

2. Add the remaining ingredients to the bowl and toss with a fork and spoon until everything is evenly coated in dressing. Taste and adjust the seasoning and serve right away, or refrigerate for up to an hour or so.

*Note: You can replace the veggies in this bowl with whatever is seasonally available. If winter, use squash and kale. There is a recipe for a quinoa bowl with winter veggies on AgelessDietLife.com.

Grain Bowl

(serves 4)

Salt, as needed

2/3 cup uncooked red or white quinoa, well rinsed

2/3 cup uncooked brown or black rice

2 tablespoons soy sauce

4 teaspoons finely chopped or grated peeled ginger

1 tablespoon rice wine or apple cider vinegar

¼ cup toasted sesame oil

1 large stalk of broccoli, steamed, stalk and florets cut into bite-
sized chunks

4 large eggs (or to make vegan: 1 cup edamame, blanched)

1 avocado, peeled, pitted and sliced

3 radishes, thinly sliced

1 cup coarsely chopped kimchi or pickles (choose naturally fermented ones, like Bubbies)

Sliced scallions (about 4), green and white parts, for serving

Sesame seeds, for serving

Crumbled dried seaweed snack sheets or nori (about 2 for each
person), for serving

1. Bring a large pot of well-salted water to a boil and add quinoa
(for 2/3 to 1 cup of quinoa, add 2 cups of water). Cover pot and
let simmer over low heat for 15-20 minutes. Turn off the heat
and let rest, covered, for 5 minutes longer. Fluff the quinoa with
a fork.

2. Do the same with the brown or black rice, cooked in well-salted
water for about 25-30 minutes (for 2/3 to 1 cup rice, add 2 cups
of water).

3. In a small bowl, whisk together soy sauce, freshly grated ginger, vinegar and salt to taste. Whisk in the sesame oil. (You can also use 1/4 cup peanut or grapeseed oil with a teaspoon of sesame oil.)

4. Place a steamer basket in a large pot filled with an inch or two of water. Place broccoli in basket. Cover pot and cook over medium heat until broccoli is tender, about 5-7 minutes. You can also use kale instead of broccoli, simply cook the same way as the broccoli.

5. Meanwhile, bring a medium pot filled with water to a boil. Using a slotted spoon, carefully lower eggs into water; boil 6 minutes. Transfer eggs immediately to a bowl of ice water to cool. If vegan, blanch edamame.

6. Put a cup of quinoa/brown or black rice in each of the 4 bowls. Divide the broccoli among the bowls, mounding it on top of the rice. Arrange avocado slices next to the broccoli. Peel eggs and cut in half; place two halves on top of each bowl. Sprinkle each bowl with fermented kimchi or, my favorite, chopped *Bubbie's* pickles, sliced radishes, scallions, sesame and seaweed. Spoon soy-ginger dressing over bowls. (Or make enough for 4, and eat the rest later in the week for lunch or a quick dinner.)

Bistro Salad

(serves 4)

SALAD

1 head of broccoli, cut into small florets

2 cups of sliced mushrooms

¼ cup olive oil

Fresh lemon juice (about 1/2 a lemon)

Sea salt

Freshly ground pepper

2 garlic cloves, grated

4 large eggs

1½ pounds frisée and/or arugula, cut or torn into bite-size pieces, washed

5 tablespoons mustard vinaigrette (below)

MUSTARD VINAIGRETTE

4 tablespoons whole grain or Dijon mustard

3 tablespoons unfiltered apple cider vinegar

1/2 cup olive oil

Sea salt

Freshly ground pepper

1. Preheat oven to 450°. Toss carrots, squash, and broccoli with oil, grated garlic and season with salt and pepper. Arrange in a single layer on a rimmed baking sheet. Roast, rotating pans halfway through, until vegetables are tender, 20–25 minutes.

2. On another smaller baking sheet roast the mushrooms with olive oil, salt, pepper, and a smaller amount of garlic for about 12 minutes.

3. Place roasted vegetables in a large bowl with 3 tablespoons of fresh lemon juice (about 1/2 a lemon), and toss to combine. Reserve 3 cups roasted vegetables for tomorrow's lunch.

4. Make the dressing, whisking all the ingredients together. Season to taste with salt and pepper.

5. Poach the eggs. Fill a saucepan with a couple inches of water. Bring the water to a boil and then lower the heat until the water is at a gentle simmer. Cook the eggs one at a time, crack the egg into a small bowl. Gently slip the egg into the water. You can use a spoon to push the egg whites closer to their yolks, to help them hold together, if you want. Wait about 30 seconds to add the next egg to the saucepan, keeping some distance between them. Cook for about 3 minutes, until the whites are opaque and cooked through and yolks are still runny. Use a slotted spoon to remove the eggs from the water, dry on a towel, and serve almost immediately.

6. Toss frisée and/or arugula and roasted vegetables with mustard vinaigrette and season with sea salt and pepper. Divide salad among plates and top each with a poached egg. Garnish the egg with sea salt and pepper.

Butternut Squash Chickpea Salad

(serves 2-4)

1 (15 oz.) can of chickpeas, rinsed and drained

1 bunch of mint, chopped or torn

Juice from 1 lemon

1/4 cup extra-virgin olive oil

1 medium butternut squash, peeled, seeded, and cut into
  1 1/2-inch pieces

1 pound Brussels sprouts, cored and halved

1 yellow or orange bell pepper, diced

1 bunch of wild arugula, torn into pieces

Sea salt and fresh pepper, to taste

1. Preheat the oven to 425°. On a baking sheet toss the butternut squash with tablespoon of olive oil and a pinch of salt. Roast for 25 minutes, or until soft. Remove from the oven and cool. Squeeze juice from 1/2 a lemon over squash, toss to coat, and season with salt.

2. Once the squash is done turn the oven down to Preheat oven to 350°. Place Brussels sprouts in a cast iron frying pan (or a roasting pan). Toss with 1/2 tablespoon oil so that the sprouts are well coated. Sprinkle generously with salt (at least a half teaspoon). Cook for about 20-25 minutes.

3. In a large bowl whisk together juice from 1/2 a lemon and the rest of the olive oil. Season with about 1/2 teaspoon of salt.

4. Add the chickpeas, squash, Brussels sprouts, and bell pepper. Toss until coated with the dressing. Add have the arugula and all the mint. Toss the salad until everything is coated. Serve salad over the rest of the arugula, drizzle a little more olive oil and season, to taste, with salt and pepper

Chinese Chicken Salad
(serves 4-6)

DRESSING

1/4 cup peanut or safflower oil

3 tablespoons toasted sesame oil

1/4 cup fresh lime juice

1/4 cup tamari (or gluten-free soy sauce)

1/4 rice wine vinegar

2 teaspoons fish sauce (such as nam pla or nuoc nam)

3 tablespoons freshly grated peeled ginger

1 tablespoon chili-garlic paste

SALAD

1 small head of red cabbage or Napa cabbage, thinly sliced
  (about 5 cups)

2 stalks celery, thinly sliced

1 small red bell pepper, thinly sliced

1 small yellow bell pepper, thinly sliced

2 medium carrots, peeled, shredded

6 scallions, whites and pale greens only, thinly sliced

3 cups shredded rotisserie or leftover chicken

2 hearts of romaine lettuce, thinly sliced

1/3 cup chopped fresh cilantro

1/2 cup chopped roasted cashews

(Optional) 14 ounces of shirataki noodles, cooked

1. Whisk the ingredients for the dressing together in a large bowl.

2. Add cabbage, carrots, scallions, bell pepper, celery, chicken, lettuce, and cilantro; toss to coat.

3. If using shirataki noodles: cook according to instructions on the package. (The cooking process takes less than 5 minutes.) Once cooked, drizzle with a little sesame oil.

4. Serve salad over the noodles. Top with cashews.

Fresh Herbs and Mushroom Omelet
(serves 4)

3 tablespoons extra-virgin olive oil

1/3 a large white or yellow onion (about 2/3 a cup), minced

5 large white, shiitake, or cremini mushrooms, rinsed briefly and wiped dry, sliced

Sea salt

Freshly ground pepper to taste

1 cup of fresh herbs (3/4 cup for the omelet, the rest for garnish), minced right before using - parsley, basil, chervil work well

6 eggs

1 teaspoon dried oregano

1/2 teaspoon dried thyme

1/2 teaspoon cumin

1. Heat the olive oil over medium-high heat in a heavy 10 or 12-inch skillet. (I like to use a well-seasoned cast-iron skillet.) Add the cumin, thyme, oregano, and a teaspoon of salt. When the oil is hot, add the onions, sauté until softened and almost golden, about 5 minutes, add the mushrooms, cook, stirring or tossing often, until they begin to sweat and soften, 3-5 minutes. Add the fresh herbs, stir until wilted, less than a minute.

2. Beat the room temperature eggs in a large bowl (you can do this while the mushrooms are cooking). Add a couple of tablespoons of water to the eggs and keep beating. This will make them frothier and lighter.

3. Pour the eggs over the mushroom, herb mixture. Distribute the eggs and the mushrooms evenly in the skillet with a spatula. Allow to cook over medium-high heat for the first few minutes. Once a few layers of egg have cooked turn the heat down to low, cook unattended about 25 minutes.

4. After 25 minutes, flip the eggs. Be bold, if the omelet breaks in half, put it back together, once flipped. Cook for another 2-3 minutes. Remove from heat. Allow to cool for about 3 minutes. Carefully flip the omelet onto a platter, the bottom side up, chop the remaining fresh herbs and scatter over the omelet, drizzle a little olive oil over it, and serve, cutting into wedges. This is delicious whether hot, warm, or cold. Serve with a green salad.

*Notes:*I find the eggs easier to crack and beat when they're at room temperature. With fresh herbs, also chop or tear (if it's basil, tear), at the last minute, right before using. For this particular dish, I used basil and parsley, but any combination of herbs you love will work nicely in this dish.

Ginger Soy Citrus Salmon
(serves 4)

1 pound wild caught Pacific salmon

4 inch piece of ginger, grated

1 garlic clove, grated

1/4 cup soy sauce (Nama Shoyu, preferably)

1/2 cup rice wine vinegar

1/2 lime, juiced

2 tablespoons olive oil

Sea salt

Fresh black pepper

1 scallion, green and white parts sliced on the bias, scattered over the baked salmon

1. Combine the soy sauce, rice wine vinegar, garlic and 3/4 of the ginger in a sauce pan.

2. Cook for 10 minutes, until it reduces to a thicker consistency.

3. Remove from heat and add the remaining ginger and the lime juice. Let cool.

4. Season salmon with a small pinch of sea salt and black pepper. Place salmon in a dish, skin side down. Rub the salmon with olive oil, spoon half the marinade over the salmon. Let sit for at least 10 minutes. Salmon can marinate for up to 3 hours.

5. Rub the bottom of a baking dish with olive oil and place the marinated salmon in it, skin side down. Spoon a tablespoon of the remaining marinade over the fish. Bake for 10 minutes at 250°.

6. Spoon another tablespoon of marinade over the fish and return to the oven for another 10 minutes. Continue to do this until the fish is cooked to medium rare (gives a little more resistance when you push it). Season with salt and fresh pepper, to taste.

7. Garnish with the scallions and serve.

Quinoa Tabbouleh

(serves 4-6)

1 cup quinoa, rinsed well

1/2 teaspoon sea salt, plus more to taste

1/2 teaspoon cumin

1/2 teaspoon cayenne (for a little kick, optional)

Juice from 1 lemon + 1 tablespoon of lemon zest

1 garlic clove, minced

1/2 cup extra-virgin olive oil

Freshly ground black pepper

1 large English hothouse cucumber or cut into 1/4-inch pieces

1 pint cherry tomatoes, halved or 4 organic Roma tomatoes, finely diced

1 cup chopped organic flat-leaf Italian parsley (about half a bunch of parsley)

1/2 cup chopped fresh mint

3 scallions, thinly sliced

1. Finely dice tomatoes or halve the cherry tomatoes (if it's winter, these grape or cherry tomatoes are your best bet), put in a bowl with a little sea salt and cracked pepper, gently sir. Allow to sit for the 15 minutes it takes the quinoa to cook.

2. Bring quinoa, 1 teaspoon of salt, and 1 1/2 cups water to a boil in a medium saucepan over high heat. Reduce heat to medium-low, cover, and simmer until quinoa is tender, about 10 minutes. Remove from heat and let stand, covered, for about 5 minutes.

3. Whisk lemon juice and garlic in a big bowl. Gradually whisk in olive oil. Season dressing to taste with salt and pepper.

4. Add cumin, cayenne, lemon zest, cucumber, tomatoes, herbs, and scallions to the bowl with the dressing, toss to coat. Add the

quinoa to the mixture and gently combine quinoa until every component of the salad is dressed. Season to taste with salt and pepper.

Note: If you want, you can add wild-caught salmon, making this a very hearty supper (or lunch). Buy a can of sustainably caught, Pacific salmon. Flake the salmon over the tabbouleh, drizzle a little extra olive oil and lemon juice.

Black Beans and Brown Rice

(serves 4-6)

2 cups organic short-grain brown rice, cooked (1/2 cup cooked rice per person) *1/2 cup of uncooked rice equals 1 cup cooked

2 cans black beans, drained and rinsed

3 cloves garlic, minced

1/2 white onion, finely diced

1 jalapeno pepper, seeded and chopped

1 pasilla or poblano pepper, chopped

1/2 bunch cilantro, chopped (or more if you want, cilantro is a wonderful anti-inflammatory herb)

2-3 medium-sized organic tomatoes, coarsely chopped

2 tablespoons avocado or olive oil

1 teaspoon sea salt

1/4 teaspoon cayenne, optional

1 teaspoon cumin

1/2 teaspoon ground coriander

1 teaspoon smoked paprika or ground chipotle

1 teaspoon Mexican oregano

1 tablespoon organic, unfiltered apple cider vinegar

2 organic limes

Olive oil

Juice from 1/2 lemon

1 bunch organic red leaf lettuce torn in bite-sized pieces

2 organic avocado, cut in chunks

Organic sprouts, alfalfa, radish, broccoli, or your favorite

1. In a cast-iron pan add avocado or olive oil and the dried spices and salt, heat it over a medium flame, when it's hot, add the onion and jalapeno. Sauté till the onion is cooked; add the garlic, sauté for a few minutes more, combining all the ingredients. Add the tomato and the cilantro. Sauté for 2 minutes, and then add the beans. Cook for a minute, gently stirring the beans, careful not to mash them, and then add the pasilla/poblano pepper. Cook another 5 minutes, until all the ingredients meld together. Add a splash of apple cider vinegar; stir the mixture, and a squeeze of a lime, for brightness. Stir again and then remove from the heat.

2. While the black beans sit, prepare a quick guacamole. Take the 2 avocados, chop them in chunky pieces, keeping it rustic, add the juice from 1 lime, a teaspoon of salt, and a little of the cilantro left over. Using a fork, gently stir the ingredients together, taking care to keep the chunks of avocado intact. I like it chunky and simple. Lots of lime, lots of avocado. Add the juice from the other half of the remaining lime if you need it. If you prefer, you can skip the quick guacamole and serve the black beans and rice with slices of avocado.

3. Dress the greens with a little olive oil, citrus (I prefer lemon, but lime will do), and salt, toss together. If you're skipping the guacamole, then add 1/2 chopped avocado to your green salad.

4. Serve the black beans over a half cup of brown rice (or a sweet potato) in a big bowl. On top of that add the dressed greens, then the guacamole, and alfalfa (or your favorite) sprouts, and enjoy!

Shredded Chicken Tacos
(serves 4)

1 15 oz. can of black beans, drained and rinsed

1 green onion, white and green parts, chopped

1/2 teaspoon ground cumin

Pinch of sea salt

1 teaspoon freshly ground pepper

2 cups of shredded chicken, seasoned with a salt, pepper, and (optional) vinegary hot sauce

3-4 leaves of lettuce, shredded

1 cucumber, finely diced

2 avocados, sliced

Sprouts (alfalfa, sunflower, radish, broccoli)

Apple cider vinegar

Extra-virgin olive oil

8 corn tortillas

Lime wedges, for serving

Hot sauce, optional

Salsa, for serving

1. Drain and rinse the beans and add them to a saucepan over low heat and warm through. Add about 1/4 cup water, the green onion, cumin, salt, and pepper and mash a large fork until coarsely mashed but not entirely smooth. Taste for salt and pepper, then turn off the heat and keep covered until needed.

2. Preheat the oven to 400°. Brush the tops of the tortillas with a bit of olive oil and lay them on a rimmed baking sheet (it's fine if they overlap). Bake until just lightly browned, 6-8 minutes. Remove from the oven and set aside.

3. Dress the lettuce and diced cucumber with a tablespoon of olive oil, a small splash of vinegar, salt, and pepper.

4. Season the shredded chicken with a little vinegary hot sauce (optional), pinch of salt and pepper.

5. Top each tortilla with a spoonful of the bean mash, about a 1/4 cup of shredded chicken, lettuce/cucumber mixture, sprouts, sliced avocado, garnish with lime wedge, and serve with salsa and hot sauce.

David's Yucatan-Style Black Bean Tacos
(serves 4)

2 15 oz. cans of organic black beans, drained and rinsed

1/2 white onion, finely diced

1 clove of garlic, minced

1 large carrot, finely diced

1 stalks of celery, finely diced

1 jalapeño, finely diced

2 tablespoons olive oil

Sea salt and pepper

1 teaspoon ground cumin

1/2 lime juiced

8-10 corn tortillas warmed

Guacamole

Sprouts

Lime wedges, for serving

1. Preheat oven to 350°, take a large sheet of foil and place the tortillas on it, wrap them, and put them in the oven to warm.

2. Place a pan on medium high heat, add 2 tablespoons olive oil, 1/2 teaspoon of salt, and cumin. Once oil is shimmering with heat, add the onions, sauté until softened, add the garlic and jalapeño. Sauté until garlic is fragrant, about a minute. Add the carrots and celery, and continue to cook, until they are tender, about 5 minutes. Add the black beans. Cook for another 2 minutes. Add the lime juice, continue to cook another minute, and then remove from heat. Season to taste with salt and pepper.

3. Take the tortillas out of the oven.

4. Serve the tacos on warm tortillas, top with the black bean mixture and sprouts, serve with lime wedges and guacamole.

Roasted Chicken
(serves 4)

3 tablespoons olive oil, divided

1 3½–4-lb. pasture-raised, organic chicken

Kosher salt and freshly ground black pepper

1 lemon, cut in half

Fresh herbs (rosemary, thyme, oregano), if you have

1. Preheat oven to 425°. Heat 1 tablespoon olive oil in a large oven-proof skillet over medium-high. Season chicken inside and out with salt and pepper, and cook, breast side down, until golden brown. Use tongs to gently rotate chicken, careful not to tear skin, and brown on all sides, 12–15 minutes total.

2. Stuff both halves of lemon and fresh herbs in the cavity, drizzle remaining olive oil over chicken. Place it, breast side up, put it in the oven.

3. Roast until an instant-read thermometer inserted into the thickest part of chicken thigh registers 165°, 35–40 minutes. If you don't have a thermometer, check doneness by cutting into thigh meat right at the joint. If the juices run clear, the bird is ready.

4. Allow chicken to rest at least 15 minutes before carving.

Fresh Tomato & Lentil Soup with Herbs

(serves 4-6, or make for 1 and have leftovers all week)
Perfect dish for summer or winter. This dish gets better each day, and there will be enough left over for a lunch.

2 tablespoons of olive oil + more to drizzle

1 large white onion, finely diced

3-4 cloves of garlic, minced

1-3 cups dried red lentils

1 teaspoon dried basil

1 teaspoon dried thyme

1 teaspoon dried oregano

1 jalapeno, diced (if you like a little hit of heat)

1 teaspoon Spanish smoked paprika (if you want a little smokiness, if you want it fresher tasting, skip the paprika)

Sea salt

6 big ripe tomatoes (if they're in season), blanched, peeled, chopped, or two 28 oz. cans whole peeled tomatoes chopped with liquid

1/2 cup fresh basil + more for garnish

1/2 cup fresh Italian herbs (like flat-leaf parsley, oregano, thyme, and marjoram)

Juice from 3-4 lemons

Vegetable Stock (one container, 32 oz.)

Braggs Liquid Aminos or tamari, to taste (about 2-3 tablespoons)

1. In a big saucepot, heat olive oil over medium heat, sauté onion with a 1/2 teaspoon of sea salt for 4-5 minutes, until almost translucent, then add garlic, jalapeno, dried herbs and spices, sauté for about 5 minutes.

2. Add lentils, sauté for about 3 minutes.

3. Add the tomatoes (if using fresh, blanch them, peel them, slice them before adding them to this mixture, if canned add the tomatoes, chopped, with the liquid), stir for about a minute, add lemon juice, salt, heat to boiling, and simmer for 5 minutes, stirring occasionally.

4. Add the fresh herbs, chopped, stir, and then add the vegetable broth, simmer for about 30 minutes.

5. Salt and pepper to taste.

6. Garnish with more fresh basil and/or parsley and drizzle a little EVOO. I often top this with fresh arugula too and serve over brown rice.

*Note: No need to pre-soak the dried lentils; they'll soften as they cook. Use 1 cup if you want more of a soup consistency and use 2 cups if you prefer a stew-like dish. Use 3 cups if you want to highlight the lentils in the soup versus the tomatoes. I like a thicker consistency and often eat it with brown rice or another whole grain so I'll use 3 or more cups.

Vegan Nori Roll

(serves 1)

1 sheet nori

2 tablespoons tahini

1/4 cup kaiware sprouts

1/4 cup mung bean sprouts

1/4 cup shredded carrots

1/2 small cucumber, cut into matchsticks

1/4 avocado, sliced thinly

1 tablespoon nutritional yeast flakes

Fresh lime juice

Sea salt, to taste

1. Arrange the nori sheet on a cutting board or bamboo sushi mat with the long edge close to you.

2. Spread the tahini in a thin layer over the nori sheet.

3. Sprinkle the nutritional yeast flakes over the tahini.

4. Layer the shredded carrots, cucumber sticks, bean sprouts, avocado, and kaiware sprouts on top of the bottom one-third of the nori sheet.

5. Spritz with lime juice and season with sea salt to taste.

6. Gently but firmly, roll the edge closest to you—filled with veggies—toward the center of the nori wrap, carefully rolling a sushi-like roll, using a napkin or bamboo mat to help with rolling.

7. With a sharp (serrated) knife, carefully slice the roll, serve immediately, and enjoy!

Salmon Nori Roll
(serves 1)

1 sheet of nori

2 slices of wild caught smoked salmon, trout, or baked tofu

1/2 avocado, sliced

2-3 tablespoons of carrot, radish sauerkraut, kimchi, or pickles (or your favorite naturally fermented vegetable)

1/4 cup sprouts (kaiware, radish, or alfalfa sprouts) or micro-greens

1 lime, halved

SESAME DIPPING SAUCE

1 tablespoon tamari or soy sauce

1 tablespoon apple cider vinegar

1 tablespoon toasted sesame oil

1/4 teaspoon cayenne, to taste

1. Lay a nori sheet out on a flat surface or bamboo mat

2. Top with smoked salmon.

3. Top with thin slices of avocado, kimchi, pickle, (or fermented veggie of your choice), and micro greens or sprouts. Spritz with lime juice.

4. Carefully roll the seaweed up.

5. To seal the nori sheet rub a little bit of water on the edge.

6. Whisk together the tamari, vinegar, sesame oil, and cayenne.

7. Slice the roll with a very sharp knife and serve with the dipping sauce.

CHAPTER 44

THE BIG FAT AGELESS DIET SHOPPING LIST

*"By shopping at a farmers market, you support
local agriculture, which has a great many benefits.
You keep farmers in your community. You support
a lot of values when you shop at the farmers market."*
—MICHAEL POLLAN

This is the big, fat *comprehensive* shopping list to use the whole time you're living ageless. It's a long list of anti-inflammatory foods—really tasty fruits, vegetables, grains, nuts and seeds, and lean proteins. You don't need to go out and get all of the ingredients at once. But you will want to stock up on the basics before you begin the *Reset* (please review Week One shopping list, preceding the meal plan section).

The Basics will include spices like cumin, cinnamon, turmeric, oregano, cayenne, coriander, paprika, and any other spice you love, for me that would be cumin. I love it in almost everything. Stock up regularly on fresh herbs, including parsley, cilantro, basil, and mint. And don't forget the staples, cans of chickpeas, black beans, and other legumes you enjoy, and cans of wild-caught tuna and salmon (limit your consumption to 1-2 times a month) are handy to have around, as are organic, additive-free smoked salmon and trout. And, I buy a couple of pounds of grass-fed beef and keep it in the freezer. Extra-firm, organic tofu is also good to have on hand. Check out your freezer section and load up on frozen organic berries and shelled edamame beans. Get yourself a great olive oil, coconut oil, sesame oil, sunflower oil (or another high-heat oil), tahini, and balsamic, rice wine, and apple cider vinegars. You'll also want a good gluten-free soy sauce or tamari. It's an easy way to add flavor. Nutritional yeast is also good for boosting flavor. I also always have hot sauces around. Worcestershire sauce is useful as well, especially for roasting chickens and marinating meats. A few pounds of brown and black rice, quinoa, and amaranth can be used because they're all gluten-free, especially this first week. And, then of course there's the fresh produce. You'll want kale, pears, oranges, lettuces, arugula, lemons, limes, garlic, onions, apples, avocados, sweet potatoes, sprouts, microgreens, and anything else you really love to eat.

The Big, Fat Ageless Diet Shopping List

Meats & Protein

Beef—only 100% grass-fed

Lamb—only 100% grass-fed

Bison—only 100% grass-fed

Chicken, turkey, and all other poultry—only organic, pasture-raised

Eggs—only organic, cage free, pasture-raised

Tofu—only organic, non-GMO

Wild game (from a source you know and trust)

Note: Most grocery and health food stores sell non-GMO, organic, pasture-raised eggs, pasture-raised turkey and chicken, grass-fed beef, and occasionally wild game, but you can also order it online. Eatwild.com is a good source for this.

Fish and Shellfish—wild and sustainably caught fish is best

Anchovies

Cod

Halibut

Mackerel

Mussels

Oysters

Salmon (only Pacific, wild-caught salmon, and less than twice a month, the radiation in the Pacific Ocean is quite high now)

Sardines (canned in olive oil)

Scallops

Shrimp

Tuna (use sparingly as tuna is high in mercury & only buy line-caught, wild tuna, packed in olive oil. Keep your consumption of tuna to twice a month, unless you have been tested with high mercury content in your blood, and then skip all tuna)

Fruits (if I'm missing some of your favorite fresh fruits, add them!)

(fresh, frozen, dried, and only organic)

Acai

Apples

Apricots

Avocados

Bananas

Blueberries

Blackberries

Cantaloupe

Cherries

Tart cherries

Figs

Goji Berries

Gooseberries

Kiwi

Honeydew Melon

Lemon & Lime (great for salad dressings)

Litchis or lychees

Mangoes

Melons

Oranges

Nectarines

Papayas

Peaches

Pears

Pineapples

Pomegranate

Plums

Raspberries

Strawberries

Note: I like to buy frozen organic berries (especially blueberries, raspberries, blackberries) year round and use them in smoothies or in sugar-free desserts.

Grains & Seeds

Amaranth

Buckwheat

Millet

Quinoa

Teff

Brown, Wild, Black Rice (love this rice, with it's complex nutty taste, and it's very good for you)

Kamut (after the first 28 days, and only if you're not allergic to gluten)

Farro (after the first 28 days, and only if you're not allergic to gluten)

Barley (after the first 28 days, and only if you're not allergic to gluten)

Freekeh (after the first 28 days, and only if you're not allergic to gluten or wheat, freekeh is green wheat)

Oatmeal (steel cut)

Grains with Gluten: wheat (including spelt, kamut, Einkorn, farro, durum, bulgur, semolina, and freekeh), barley, rye, triticale (a hybrid of wheat)

Gluten-free Grains: amaranth, buckwheat, corn, Job's Tears (also known as hato mugi, adlay and coix, is a member of the grass family and popular in Asian cultures as a food source), millet, montina (Indian rice grass), oats (steel-cut and rolled, oats are inherently gluten-free, but are often processed in plants that process wheat), quinoa, rice (brown, black or forbidden, wild-grain), sorghum, teff

Herbs and Spices (fresh and dried)

Allspice

Basil

Bay leaf

Cayenne

Celery Seed

Chervil

Chives

Cilantro

Cinnamon

Coriander

Cumin

Dill

Fennel

Garlic

Ginger

Marjoram

Mustard (dry)

Nutmeg

Oregano

Paprika

Parsley

Pepper (black or red)

Peppermint

Rosemary

Saffron

Sage

Savory

Tarragon

Thyme

Turmeric

Legumes, Nuts, and Seeds

Almonds

Almond butter

Adzuki beans

Black beans

Chia seeds

Chickpeas (garbanzo beans)

Flaxseeds (and meal)

Hempseeds

Hazelnuts (filberts)

Kidney beans

Lentils (red, green, black)

Lima beans or butter beans

Macadamia nuts

Navy beans

Pecans

Pine nuts

Pinto beans

Pistachios

Pumpkin seeds

Sesame seeds

Soybeans/edamame (organic only)

Sunflower seeds

Tahini (sesame seed paste)

Walnuts

If I have time, I like to sprout my legumes and nuts, makes for easier digestion, overnight. If you're sprouting your legumes and nuts, change the water several times a day & cover with something like a cheesecloth. Almonds are great to sprout too. Black beans and chickpeas take the longest, so if you're using them for a bean soup, black beans and rice, or hummus, I recommend soaking them overnight. Another trick with chickpeas is to soak them with a teaspoon of baking soda (buy all-natural, preservative-free baking soda). If I want a quick meal, I'll use canned beans.

Oils (all oils cold-pressed, organic)

Avocado Oil

Coconut oil

Extra-virgin olive oil (EVOO)

Grape seed oil

Hemp Oil

Pumpkin (seed) oil

Sesame seed oil

Sunflower oil

Walnut oil

Vegetables (if I missed your favorite fresh vegetables, add yours to this list)

Alfalfa sprouts

Arugula

Asparagus

Basil

Beets (beet greens, the tops of beets are great cooked, in smoothies, in omelets, and stir fries)

Bell peppers (green, red, orange, or yellow)

Bok choy

Broccoli

Brussels sprouts

Cabbage (green, red, Napa, or Savoy)

Carrots

Chinese cabbage

Collards

Daikon radish (greens are great to use as well in stir-fries and soups)

Dandelion greens

Endive (great in salads)

Escarole (even better for you & better tasting than green & red leaf lettuces)

Fennel

Green beans

Kale (Lacinato, Tuscan, red, green)

Kohlrabi

Leeks

Lettuce (green and red leaf, romaine, baby gem, butter)

Mung Beans (great in nori rolls, tacos, salads, and stir-fries)

Microgreens

Mushrooms (all mushrooms are great, especially wild and shii-take)

Mustard greens (turnip greens are good to eat too!)

Onions (green, red, white, or yellow)

Peas & pea shoots

Radicchio

Radishes

Scallions

Sea vegetables (seaweed, kelp)

Spinach

Squash (summer or winter, butternut, buttercup, kabocha, acorn, etc.)

Sweet potatoes

Swiss chard

Tomatoes

Turnips

Watercress

Recommended Products

Bubbies pickles

Nama Shoyu soy sauce (it's fermented and organic, though not always gluten free, so check the label)

Braggs Liquid Aminos

Alvarado St. Bakery sourdough bread

Miscellaneous Items

Nori

Nutritional yeast flakes

White miso paste

Unfiltered apple cider vinegar

Dark chocolate (at least 70% cocoa with 5g or less sugar per serving)—no chocolate though for the first 6 weeks

Naturally fermented, pickled foods (kimchi, sauerkraut, miso, pickles, soy sauce, and vegetables)

Organic or biodynamic red wine

Dark beer (pale ales, IPAs, porters, stouts)

Tea (green, white, or black)

Sprouted, organic corn tortillas (these are terrific for making wraps or soft tacos for lunch)

Worcestershire sauce and hot sauces (great for brightening a dish and imparting a little heat)

Maca powder (maca is from a root found in Perú, it's a powerful adaptogenic and many consider it a superfood)

Bee pollen (made by honey bees, it's the food of the young bee, and is widely considered a superfood, it's rich in proteins, vitamins, including B-complex, folic acid, and it's good in smoothies)

The top three allergens. These are not part of the Ageless Diet and they are inflammatory. Eliminate these from your diet for at least 6 weeks:

1. Sugar
2. Dairy
3. Wheat

AND eliminate all processed foods (these include cheeses, chips, corn products, sauces, pre-packaged meals, cereals, fast food, mayonnaise, ketchup, artificial sweeteners & sugar substitutes, sodas, margarine, all foods labeled diet, low-calorie, yogurt, etc.).

The Breakdown:
• Foods to eliminate for 6 weeks: processed foods, almost all dairy, all added sugar (in any and all things), artificial sweeteners, sugar substitutes, most wheat and breads.

• After the first 3 weeks you can reintroduce very small amounts of dairy, and only grass-fed. Observe how you feel, if it's an allergen for you. But I highly recommend you give up dairy most of the time, except for small quantities of goat milk dairy.

• After 28 days, slowly reintroduce some grains and whole wheat, noticing how you feel, if you have an allergic reaction. Reintroduction of grains will include oats, rye, spelt, farro, barley, freekeh, etc.

• For the full 6 weeks: no added sugar of any kind (and if you go the full six weeks with no sugar, why not continue with a sugar free diet? don't hop back on that sugar train).

Ageless Diet *Cleanse* (the first 7 Days)

MONDAY—SUNDAY
AM Smoothie
Lunch
PM Smoothie
Dinner
No food after 6:00 p.m.

Ageless Diet *Reset*

Pre-*Reset*	The Week Before 6-Week *Reset* + 7-Day *Cleanse*
1	Order all supplements for the *Cleanse* + *Reset*
2	Check out new exercise classes you want to try, find a meditation you think you'll enjoy, do a little fun research for activities you'll want to do during the *Reset*
3	Make room in your schedule this coming week for daily 30-minute workouts, 12-minute meditations, and a good night's sleep
4	Clean out kitchen—get rid off all junk foods, sugar, dairy, processed wheat (if junk food isn't around you won't eat it)
5	Stock your kitchen with healthy foods (if you're not hungry enough for an apple, you're not really hungry)
6	Shop for the first week's meal plan—get the basics, smoothie fixings, fruits and vegetables to snack on
7	On Sunday before you begin Day 1 of *Cleanse*: Do meal plan prep—chop veggies for salads, roast chicken (if you're roasting one), roast veggies, make salad dressings

Week 1	**The *Cleanse***
1	Drop the Big 3: Dairy, Wheat (and grains with gluten), Sugar (all added sugars and sugar substitutes)
2	No alcohol for the first 7 days
3	No coffee for the first 7 days
4	No food after 6:00 p.m. (eat your last meal of the day before 6:00 p.m.)
5	2 Detox Smoothies—one in the morning and one in the afternoon
6	Eat mostly vegan (aim for a 70-80% vegan diet)
7	Take the supplements (source the right ones, use AgelessDietLife.com as a guide, if you're uncertain about where to find the right, high-quality supplements)
Note	Make sure to take the supplements at the appropriate times, especially the serotonin-support sleep supplements (take them 30 minutes before bedtime)

Week 2	**The *Reset***
1	Coffee (organic, free-trade) is allowed, no coffee after 2:00 p.m. though
2	Limit all alcohol consumption to wine (organic or biodynamic), no more than 2 glasses
3	No dairy
4	No wheat
5	No added sugars
6	You can eat after 6:00 p.m., if you want
7	Continue taking the supplements, meal planning, and food prepping, keep the kitchen stocked with ageless-approved foods, stay away from junk

Week 3	**The *Reset***
1	Try new workouts
2	Keep meditating daily
3	Keep up with the supplements
4	No dairy, no wheat, no added sugar, no processed foods
5	Keep the kitchen stocked with healthy foods

Week 4	**The *Reset***
1	You may add back a little dairy (try sticking with goat milk dairy, it's easier to digest), add it back in limited amounts
2	No wheat (and no grains with gluten), no added sugars, no processed foods

Week 5	**The *Reset***
1	You may add back grains containing gluten, but stay away from "modern" dwarf wheat, processed wheat, and processed foods containing wheat
2	If you're not gluten-intolerant, you may add beer (preferably darker beer from micro-brewery)
3	No added sugars, no processed foods
4	Keep up with supplements, meditation, and exercise

Week 6	**The *Reset***
1	Try new workouts
2	Keep meditating daily
3	Keep up with the supplements
4	NO processed foods, no added sugars (Explore new foods, new whole grains, new recipes)